GET

YOUR BODY

BACK

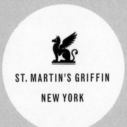

ST. MARTIN'S GRIFFIN
NEW YORK

GET YOUR BODY BACK

Lose Weight,
Gain Energy, and
Get Fit After
Having Your Baby

ANITA WEIL BELL

www.stmartins.com

Book design by Gretchen Achilles

Library of Congress Cataloging-in-Publication Data

Bell, Anita Weil.
    Get your body back : lose weight, gain energy, and get fit after having your baby / Anita Weil Bell.—1st St. Martin's Griffin ed.
        p.   cm.
Includes bibliographical references (p. 231).
    ISBN 0-312-28339-3
    1. Postnatal care.   2. Physical fitness for women.   I. Title.
    RG801.B229   2002
    618.6—dc21   2002003647

FIRST EDITION: OCTOBER 2002

10   9   8   7   6   5   4   3   2   1

NOTE TO READERS

The dietary recommendations, meal plans, exercises, program, and advice in this book are in no way intended as a substitute for medical consultation. We urge the reader to consult with her doctor before beginning this diet or program or any regimen of exercise. This program is not intended for women with any illnesses or other conditions that may be worsened by an unsupervised diet or exercise program. The author and publisher disclaim any liability or loss, personal or otherwise, resulting from the dietary recommendations, meal plans, exercises, program, or advice in this book. Some of the names in the anecdotes have been changed to afford the individuals privacy.

CONTENTS

PART ONE

THE INGREDIENTS OF
WEIGHT LOSS AND FITNESS

PART TWO

THE GET YOUR BODY BACK PROGRAM

ACKNOWLEDGMENTS

Thanks to my editor at St. Martin's Press, Heather Jackson, a talented professional and world-class mommy. Heather had the idea for this book after the birth of her adorable son, Louis. Now Louis is running around, charming everyone he meets, and Heather looks better than ever.

As always, thanks to my wonderful agent, Faith Hamlin. Faith combines the best attributes of a strong businesswoman and a caring mom, just what every author needs.

Many thanks also to Ed Prestwood of CyberSoft, Inc., creator of Nutribase Software, for providing an outstandingly helpful, comprehensive, user-friendly tool.

Much love to my mother, Shirley Weil, and my father, Gilbert Weil. Now in their seventies and married over fifty years, they epitomize the potential for lifelong love and fitness.

Love and thanks to my husband, Jonathan Bell, for creative recipes and unending romance. And thanks for the many times he entertained Belinda with festive suppers and after-dinner dancing so that I could write in the evenings.

Finally, thanks to my daughter, Belinda Claire Bell, for giving me the most satisfying and fascinating experience of a lifetime: motherhood. The love and joy she gives our family is beyond anything I could imagine or express.

INTRODUCTION: THE BASICS OF THE GET YOUR BODY BACK PROGRAM

The year I had my baby girl, Belinda, five other babies were born in my tiny Hudson Valley village. We six new mothers started an informal "baby club," and met once a month at each other's houses. As we watched the babies grow, it was interesting to see how our own bodies changed after childbirth. Here's how we fared:

- Lynette, a reed-slim California blonde, was back in her size 2 jeans after three months and could even flaunt a crop top with her flat stomach showing. Naturally thin, she said the weight just "fell off." She had another baby two years later and was skinny again six weeks after delivery. If she wasn't so sweet, we'd all hate her.

- Catherine, tall and athletic, weighed even less than before her pregnancy, after only two months of exclusively breast-feeding her infant. Still, she complained she wasn't as firm as before because she didn't have time to exercise.

- Jennifer kept on about 15 pounds, in her stomach and thighs. She finally lost it after following a strict diet for four months and walking her baby every day in a jogger-stroller. She was fortunate that her baby was one of those who was content in the carriage.

- Megan, who had always struggled with extra weight, had gained 60 pounds during the pregnancy and experienced gestational diabetes. Six months after delivery, she had only dropped 20 pounds. Megan tried a drastic liquid diet and lost 30 pounds in a matter of six weeks, but gained it back quickly.

- Susan, who had always maintained her moderate weight easily, lost all the pregnancy pounds without effort after having her first baby. But after having her second child (eighteen months later) she kept on an extra 15 pounds or so. She said she was eating the same way she always had, but the weight stayed.

- I gained 30 pounds during pregnancy and lost 20 pounds easily after the birth, during the first few months of intensive breast-feeding. But the last 10 pounds stubbornly stayed on for two years, even though I was eating the same as I had before childbirth. Having had Belinda when I was almost thirty-nine, I didn't know whether it was really baby fat or turning forty that accounted for my thickening figure. However, after less than two months of following the principles of the Get Your Body Back Program, those last 10 pounds were gone, I'm happy to report!

You've probably observed a similar cross section. Some women get their figures back only a few months after delivery, some take a year or two. Many are never the same again. It's hard to discern a pattern of who loses and who doesn't. Some women have the discipline to methodically reduce fat and calories and exercise regularly after having a baby. But many mommies are too tired and busy to exercise and in no frame of mind to stick with a diet. They may eat the same amount as they did before giving birth, but the weight stays put.

Each day, approximately 10,000 women deliver a baby in the United States. They range in age from teens to mid forties (and a few are even older). Their weight gain during pregnancy could be anywhere from 15 to 60 pounds, with 30 to 35 pounds the recommended median. Their ethnic and genetic predispositions run the full gamut. Yet a basic pattern prevails.

Three months after delivery, 30 percent of new moms are back to their preconception weight. Six months after delivery, approximately half the women have returned to their prebaby weight. And about one-ninth of new moms in the United States weigh *less* six months after giving birth than they did before conception.

These statistics tell you that it's possible, even probable, to get your body back after having a baby. But if you're reading this book, you probably belong to the growing group of women who do not effortlessly shed their pregnancy weight gain.

There are many reasons why you might be retaining extra weight:

- Eating more: eating more frequently, eating bigger portions

- Eating differently: eating more foods with high fat and sugar content

- Eating for emotional reasons: to counteract depression, stress, and/or anxiety

- Getting less aerobic exercise and exercise in general

- Undiagnosed thyroid disease

The Get Your Body Back Program gives you a blueprint for overcoming every one of these challenges. It offers you a three-month program with three major components:

1. The Healthy Eating Light Plan (HELP) for Moms. This plan helps you lose extra weight while maintaining high nutritional standards. The recipes use fresh, nutritious ingredients to create quick and easy meals. Seven days of different meals plans are provided for each month of the program. These meal plans are repeated each week to keep the program simple and practical. Nursing mothers will add "breastfeeding bonus foods" to provide extra nutrition for baby.

2. The Workable Workouts: Exercise routines that are realistic for the time-crunched, always tired new mom. The emphasis is on exercise you can do with your baby along. The exercise program will enhance your metabolism, increase your energy, elevate your mood, and let you regain your prepregnancy body tone.

3. Mommy Care: Overeating or wrong food choices are often linked to emotional issues, stress, and fatigue. This component of the plan gives you ways to nourish your emotional health, so you can cope with the difficulty of being a mother and fully appreciate the joy.

The primary goal of the Get Your Body Back Program is to help you return to your prepregnancy weight and level of fitness. If you follow the program, you are likely to lose 10 to 20 pounds over a three-month period. You will also firm and tone your body, and find your mood and energy level improved. If you're seeking to lose more weight or to be thinner and stronger than you were before conceiving, you can continue to follow the basic principles of the program after the three months are over.

It's best to wait until you are two to three months postpartum to embark on the program. Before that, you can get a head start by reading this book and begin implementing the principles. You can stay away from fatty foods and sweets as much as possible and begin some basic exercise when you are six weeks postpartum, if you have your doctor's approval. But it's unlikely you'll be ready to take a disciplined approach to the program for the first few months of your baby's life. Just enjoy the wonder of loving your infant, and rest and rejuvenate as much as possible.

By three months postpartum, you can assess what weight you have taken off without effort. Your baby has passed the newborn stage and should be more settled, sleeping and digesting better. You can begin (barely) to think about something other than your baby.

Even so, it's difficult to embark on a complicated diet at any time in the first few years of motherhood. That's why the meal plans are kept simple. There are no complicated food-combining formulas to master, just easy-to-prepare meal plans and sensible guidelines. You can rest assured that you're getting all the nutrition you require to be strong and healthy, with ample nourishment to pass on to your baby if you're nursing.

This is not a time in your life to experiment with cutting-edge diets or drive yourself to the edge of collapse with intense workouts. Adjusting to motherhood makes so many demands on your body and your emotions. This is a time to be good to yourself, to follow the proven principles of healthy eating.

Remember that this program is not a response to the relentless pressure to be thin. It is created to help you feel comfortable in your own body—strong, energetic, and well-nourished. The goal is to attain a physical and emotional sense of well-being, to feel your best and enjoy being a healthy mom.

NOTE TO READERS: For the sake of simplicity, this book some-times refers to "your husband." Please don't feel excluded if you are not married, if you have a female partner, or whatever your circumstances. Whether you work outside the home, stay at home with your baby, have one child or two or more children, this book is meant for you. The Get Your Body Back Program is an inclusive program intended to help *all* mothers enjoy radiant fitness.

PART ONE

THE INGREDIENTS
OF WEIGHT LOSS
AND FITNESS

CHAPTER 1

THE PRINCIPLES BEHIND THE GET YOUR BODY BACK PROGRAM

Perhaps you've tried other diet/exercise programs to take off your baby weight. Or at least you've gone as far as buying the books, watching the television shows, checking out the advice on the Internet. But you haven't been able to stay with any of the plans.

Well, who can blame you? If your baby is still waking up many times a night, you're so tired that you can barely think straight. Your hormones are fluctuating and your body is recovering in other ways. You're getting used to the emotional realities of motherhood—the incredible highs and lows that one tiny innocent baby can create throughout the course of a day (and night).

Maybe you're marooned at home with a fridge full of tempting food. Or you're stressed out from juggling work and parenthood. You don't have the freedom to relax in the ways you used to enjoy and food is a quick fix, the only indulgence available.

In addition, there's a physiological challenge. During pregnancy, high estrogen levels signal the cells to store fat instead of releasing it. The cells can stay programmed to store fat throughout the breast-feeding period and beyond. From a survival standpoint, it makes sense for a woman's body to store calories for nursing, in case of famine. But with today's cultural pressure to be thin, along with our knowledge of the health benefits of maintaining a moderate body weight, it can be a problem.

It's always hard to stay with a nutrition and exercise program.

But the first year or two of motherhood is the most difficult time. That's why the Get Your Body Back Program strives to make it as easy and safe as possible. The meal plan is not revolutionary. It uses time-tested principles of healthy eating. The workouts do not demand that you "go for the burn" or reach new heights of aerobic intensity. Best of all, they do not even require that you have a baby-sitter or relative on call. Your baby can be right there with you when you exercise. Plus, the program addresses the emotional aspects of eating, and provides better ways than bingeing to relieve stress and get satisfaction.

This is *not* the only nutrition and exercise program that will work for you. If you have the time and perseverance, there are many plans that might work. But the Get Your Body Back Program may be the one you find easiest to follow at this point in your life. The difference is that this plan is baby-friendly. It acknowledges reality: You have very little time for yourself and limited attention and energy. Your baby is always on your mind. You need a plan that matches the reality of this special time.

THE BASICS OF THE HEALTHY EATING LIGHT PLAN (HELP) FOR MOMS

There are four basic HELP rules for weight loss.

RULE #1: EAT EARLY

Most Americans eat about 70 percent of their calories in the evening. No wonder there's an epidemic of obesity!

Your metabolism is much faster in the morning and afternoon, and dramatically slows down about twelve hours after you wake up.

The later you eat, the more likely calories are to be stored as fat, instead of burned. In essence, anything you eat at night is twice as fattening. For optimal weight loss and maintenance, the goal is to finish eating by 6:30 P.M. You can also opt to save your dessert and have it later in the evening. If you're breast-feeding, have a snack around 8 P.M.

RULE #2: EAT LESS, BUT MORE FREQUENTLY

Starving yourself as a diet strategy always backfires. It will make you short-tempered and low on energy. In addition, you're more likely to go off your diet and overeat if you've been depriving yourself. And if you're breast-feeding or caring for a baby, it's not fair to either of you.

The meals in this program are designed to ensure that you are never hungry. They provides three modest meals and two snacks or "mini-meals," spaced throughout the day at two to three hour intervals. The first meal should come no more than one half hour after you wake up so you won't start the day hungry. The five meals add up to a daily calorie count of 1500 to 1600 calories. Breast-feeding moms will add 150 to 500 calories of high-protein, high-calcium bonus foods (the caloric amount depends on whether you're breast-feeding full-time or just once or twice day).

The key to eating frequently without gaining weight is to control your portions. The meal plans will leave you satisfied, not stuffed.

RULE #3: EAT LOW-FAT FOODS

It's hardly surprising—high-fat foods are most likely to become stored as fat in your fat cells. Fat is also a relatively inefficient energy source for your body. Carbohydrates are the preferred source of energy for most of your cells. Protein is the optimal building block of muscle cells.

A diet that provides a balance of carbohydrates and protein will allow you to gain strength and energy as you lose fat. You're going to need all the energy you can get to keep up with that little baby, especially when he starts crawling, walking, and running in quick succession. You'll both be better off if you limit the amount of fat you consume.

The meal plans in this book are low in fat and high in nutritional value. They emphasize protein and complex carbohydrates, which—contrary to popular belief—are not fattening if eaten in controlled portions without high-fat condiments.

RULE #4: DRINK LOTS OF WATER

In the quest for a magic diet trick, people will try almost any type of cream, pill, or potion. But in fact, there is only one diet elixir that really works—water. Water curbs your appetite, breaks down fat, flushes out toxins, and performs a host of other miracles.

Very often, we think we're hungry when we're really thirsty. Consuming lots of fresh, filtered water will help you stay in control of your appetite. This is especially true during lactation, when a woman's ravenous appetite is often a symptom of dehydration. Nursing mothers need plenty of water for rehydration, as well as optimal milk production.

During the three months of the plan, you'll be drinking water all day long. Eight glasses for nonnursing women and ten glasses for breast-feeding mothers is recommended. It will become second nature to sip a bottle of water at the playground, take a water bottle along on play dates, and keep a frequently refilled glass on your desk at work.

THE WORKABLE WORKOUTS

Whenever I was tired, stressed, or depressed during Belinda's babyhood, my sister Janette, an incredibly fit woman (with no children), would tell me to take an aerobic exercise class. Spin classes, kick boxing, aerobic salsa dancing . . . Janette was always running out to these classes, which kept her spirits up and her clothing size down.

It all sounded great—but I never went. Since my husband is a freelance cameraman/producer, I never knew when he'd be home from work and able to watch the baby. When he was available, I usually felt frantic to catch up on laundry and writing, or to succumb to the ever-present urge to nap. Belinda was too young to be left with a strange baby-sitter at a health club. And it was too extravagant and complicated to get a sitter so I could dash to class. I knew that the only way I was going to exercise was if I could do it *with* Belinda. And that's the premise of the Workable Workouts.

It's great if you can find baby-sitting coverage and go out to an exercise class or gym on a regular basis. If you have this luxury, you're probably doing it already. But if you're like the vast majority of new moms, with limitations on free time and disposable income, you're better off learning to exercise with your baby. Then you'll actually find the time to do it.

Another benefit of the Workable Workouts is flexibility. You can do these workouts at any time that's convenient for you and your baby. This is crucial, since babies have a way of throwing a monkey wrench into schedules and appointments.

I remember visiting one of my baby club friends when her son was six months old. She had gathered exercise schedules from four different dance schools, gyms, and yoga centers and pinned them neatly to her bulletin board. When I complimented her efficiency, she said, "Oh, I've had the schedules for three months now and I haven't gone to one single class. Something always comes up."

Unless you're one of the lucky few with a live-in nanny or local grandmother, you may not have much freedom in baby's first year or two. But you can still enjoy many different workouts:

- Outdoor fitness walking, the number-one exercise for new moms

- Strength-building and stretching exercises you can do at home

- Dancing around your living room

- Indoor treadmill

- Exercise videotapes

Aerobic exercise will help you control your weight by using excess calories that would otherwise be stored as fat, and by speeding up your metabolism. Establishing exercise as a healthy habit will also enable you to keep your figure after the three months of the Get Your Body Back Program. Many studies have shown that people who combine regular exercise with a moderate reduction in fat and caloric intake are the mostly likely to maintain weight loss.

In fact, if you reduce calories and fat intake without exercise, there's a risk that your body will react as if it is starving and reduce the number of calories it burns. This will make it easier to regain weight in the future.

If you lose weight through dieting alone, 25 to 50 percent of the weight lost is muscle tissue, not fat. Then if you continue to be sedentary and regain the weight, all of the regained pounds are fat and your resting metabolism falls. This makes it harder to stay trim as you age, and with each subsequent baby you carry. A vigorous exercise program will let you avoid this all-too-common syndrome.

Another benefit of the Workable Workouts is that they promote flexibility and help prevent back and neck pain, the bane of many new mothers. Holding that wonderfully chubby baby, bending over the changing table, feeding, and nursing, all wreak havoc on a mother's spine. Flexibility exercises and movement will let you realign and recover.

There's also a strong psychological component to the Workable Workouts. Aerobic exercise influences the production of brain chemicals such as norepinephrine and endorphin that affect mood. Research also suggests that the neurotransmitter serotonin becomes more readily available in the brain with systematic physical activity. The workouts will reduce your stress level, strengthen your resolve to stay on the diet plan, and alleviate the "baby blues."

If you suffer from postpartum depression, exercise can be an important element in your recovery. Researchers are finding that regular exercise can be as effective as antidepressant medication in reducing symptoms of depression, and have a faster effect. In addition, people who exercise regularly have a lower rate of relapse of depression.

There's another advantage. Exercising will provide you with more energy to keep up with your baby. When you exercise aerobically, you burn oxygen at a faster rate. In turn, your body becomes more effective at producing and storing energy. You'll be less tempted to eat sweets for a quick spurt of energy and better able to maintain a steady level of stamina.

During the program you'll learn how to structure your workouts so that they produce noticeable toning and strengthening results, speed up your metabolism, elevate your energy, and boost your self-esteem. Plus, you'll be entertaining your baby and passing the time happily, since babies love to watch people moving. And before too long, the little one will be keeping up with you and then some!

MOMMY CARE

When a woman has a baby she often forgets about pleasing herself. Everything revolves around the baby's health, happiness, and needs. To some extent, this is natural, necessary, and admirable. But you have to devote just a tiny bit of time and effort to doing something for yourself. Otherwise, resentment and frustration can build up—and often your only outlet becomes overeating.

The Mommy Care component of the program offers a structure for giving yourself a little pampering and pleasure. Each month, activities are suggested that can reduce your tension and improve your mood. These ideas are purposefully designed to be neither expensive nor time-consuming. They are simple ways to give your spirit and energy a lift, realistic for a busy mommy.

In Europe, many wealthy women go to a hydrotherapy spa for a week or two a few months after giving birth. They relax in beautiful surroundings, tone their bodies in exercise classes, have the tension kneaded away by masseurs, rejuvenate their skin with seaweed wraps, and savor light cuisine. Doesn't that sound divine? Unless you're a member of the jet set, however, this may not be an option. You're lucky if you have time to wash your hair, let alone go to a spa resort and bake in a mud bath.

Well, there is a middle ground between the luck of the leisure class and the relentless demands that most new mothers face. It's not an all-or-nothing proposition. Giving yourself brief breaks can make a big difference in your mood and self-image.

You are more than a metabolism, a collection of fat cells and muscle tissue. Your mental/emotional state has a tremendous influence on how you eat and how well equipped you will be to follow the diet in this book, or any good advice for that matter. Attention to the emotional demands of motherhood is essential for success. A little self-indulgence in a long, busy week of babycare will do both you and your whole family a world of good.

CHAPTER 2

FOOD, MOOD, AND ENERGY

It's supposed to be the happiest time of your life. And in many ways, it is. You love your little baby more than anything on earth. You're incredibly relieved that the pregnancy and birth are over. You can't stop gazing at and kissing your perfect baby. It's a pleasure to share your bundle of joy with the people you love, and even with strangers. Everyone admires a new mom and loves a little baby.

Older ladies stop you on the street, coo over the carriage, and say, "Enjoy it while they're young . . . it goes so fast." You smile and nod, but inside you may be thinking: "I do enjoy it; but I'm also exhausted and stressed out. I feel like I have no life of my own anymore and never will. Goes fast? The days and nights seem endless. What's wrong with me? This is supposed to be the happiest time of my life."

You may feel guilty, overwhelmed, deprived, dazed. You look for a little relief, a pick-me-up, in a day of endless self-sacrifice. Marooned at home, or trapped at the office, the only indulgence you find is food. So you eat too many cookies, wolf down a bag of chips, and end up feeling worse. Tired, irritable, and annoyed at yourself.

Let's be honest. The first year of a baby's life is a period of profound wonder and joy for parents. But it can also be a time of fatigue, confusion, and depression for you, the new mom. In fact, in the course of a single hour or day you can veer from elation to despair.

My husband said that he never knew who he'd find when he came home from work during that first year. The fulfilled mother, nursing in the rocking chair, gazing down at the baby blissfully. Or the overwhelmed new mom, weeping because she didn't know why the baby was crying. Or the unfair wife, berating her bewildered husband because she thought he wasn't helping enough. Does this sound familiar?

You may be one of those blessed women who easily sails through her first years of motherhood. Or you may be one of a huge contingent that has mixed emotions. Of course, you love your little baby more than anything in the world . . . that's a given. But you may not love taking care of the baby all day. Or you may be overwhelmed by juggling motherhood and other work responsibilities.

During the first year, I was in a heightened state of anxiety half the time, wondering if I was doing everything right, worrying about Belinda's precious health and safety. I felt vaguely inadequate about this response until my sister-in-law had a baby. She is a brilliant and brave emergency-room eye surgeon. Yet she said that taking care of her infant was the hardest thing she had ever done in her life. She found it more tiring and demanding than eye surgery!

There are many reasons women get depressed or have mood swings during the early stages of motherhood. A huge factor is sheer fatigue. It's doubtful that you're getting eight hours of sleep. And even if you are, it's not all in one piece. Interrupted sleep is never as restful as unbroken slumber. You may be chronically tired for the entire first year or longer.

Besides sleep disruptions and the hard work of babycare, another cause of fatigue may be an underactive thyroid gland. This common condition (discussed in more detail later in the chapter) can slow down metabolism and make it difficult to lose weight. It often strikes women after childbirth and can be mistaken for common fatigue.

Hormonal imbalances after delivery are another factor, resulting in mood swings, anxiety, and anger. While these usually resolve in the first few weeks to few months, they can linger in many cases.

Then there's working mother's guilt and ambivalence. If you go back to work, even part time, you may feel very torn. For the first two years, I had a constant feeling that I should be doing something else. When I was writing and a baby-sitter was watching Belinda, I wished I was holding my little love instead. When I spent the whole day caring for Belinda, I worried that I wasn't getting enough writing done. Like many working mothers, I constantly felt I was in the wrong place doing the wrong thing.

All of these pressures can affect your fitness level, as well as your emotional health. The two are inextricably linked. Your emotions and energy level have a tremendous influence on the choices you make regarding food and exercise. This is one reason why so many diets fail, especially during the postpartum period. The diets themselves may be sound, but you can't stick with the plan because there are underlying emotional issues.

You're tired, distracted, resentful, up and down. Your sense of discipline and will is eroded. You're devoting every ounce of strength to tending to the baby's needs and being patient with her. You have nothing left to give yourself.

Perhaps you're bored and lonely, stuck at home with the baby, and you overeat to fill the day. Feeling pleasure-deprived, you indulge in too much chocolate and ice cream. You're tired and looking for a sugar lift. Or an extra portion of pasta relaxes you.

Don't feel guilty. Be proud. You're trying to be a good mother and fulfill the endless needs of your baby. You're not deserting your family, although you may sometimes wish you could take off for Tahiti. You're not going on a drinking spree or partying all night to relieve stress. You're not blowing up at your baby when you're frustrated. You're doing the best you can. Who can blame you for snacking too much?

Eating is the most socially and morally acceptable way to seek emotional relief. It doesn't hurt your baby. It doesn't interfere with doing your duty. The nicest mothers in the world turn to food for solace. It's perfectly natural.

However, if you want to enjoy optimum energy, overcome depression, and find longer-lasting stress relief, there are better habits to develop: the right food choices instead of the wrong ones; exercise instead of lethargy, little perks that won't weigh you down. This book will give you the tools to enhance your mood and energy without negating your best intentions.

The first step is to accurately identify your current emotional state. Some new mothers think they should be blissfully happy. But the reality is that for many women this is a difficult time emotionally. It may be up and down or steadily low. This is no cause for shame. Many women worry that if they're not absolutely fulfilled by motherhood they're lacking some basic maternal instinct. This is nonsense. You can be a wonderful mother and still have mixed emotions.

POSTPARTUM DEPRESSION

Most women—an estimated eight out of ten—experience some degree of the "baby blues" in the weeks following childbirth. Crying spells, mood swings, and extreme fatigue are frequent following delivery.

For the majority of women, these symptoms ease up after a few weeks. But for many, the baby blues devolve into postpartum depression. This is far from uncommon. It is estimated that 15 to 20 percent of women experience postpartum depression that lasts beyond the first few weeks.

Any woman can develop a postpartum mood disorder. Although research indicates that there may be a hormonal component, the exact mechanisms are not fully understood. Certainly the abrupt hormonal changes following childbirth can be a factor. One of the major predictors for postpartum mood disorders is a previous experience of premenstrual mood symptoms, indicating that some women are vulnerable to hormonal fluctuations.

Another issue is the fatigue and stress involved in caring for a baby. The stress may actually alter the chemicals in the brain, resulting in serotonin deficiency and other neurotransmitter effects.

The strain that a new baby sometimes puts on a marriage can also lead to depression. Lower levels of marital satisfaction and perceived lack of support from the father are noted in many women with postpartum depression.

Ambivalence about the new role of motherhood, even in women who plan their pregnancies, is another factor. Loss of freedom and control over one's own life can precipitate depression. Women who need to be in control, who are self-critical or prone to perfectionism, may be more vulnerable.

Postpartum depression, like other forms of depression, is primarily a mood disorder that affects how we think and feel. It involves feelings of hopelessness, sadness, numbness, and a pattern of negative thinking. The ability to think rationally, concentrate, and solve problems is impaired. Physical alterations in sleep, appetite, energy, and immunity can ensue, resulting in constant fatigue and sometimes susceptibility to headache and other ailments.

The *Diagnostic and Statistical Manual* defines these symptoms for major depression:

- Depressed mood for most of the day, nearly every day
- Markedly diminished interest or pleasure in most activities
- Significant weight loss or weight gain, decrease or increase in appetite
- Insomnia (difficulty sleeping) or hypersomnia (sleeping too much)
- Agitation or slowed movements
- Fatigue or loss of energy
- Feelings of worthlessness or inappropriate guilt
- Diminished ability to think, concentrate, and make decisions
- Recurrent thoughts of death or suicide

All of these symptoms do not have to be present at once for a diagnosis of major depression. The general criteria are loss of interest or depressed mood plus four other symptoms which are present nearly every day during the same two week period, and which represent a change from previous functioning.

These criteria are only general guidelines, and professional assessment is crucial if you suspect you have depression or another mood disorder. *Do not try to diagnose yourself*, especially if you have any thoughts of suicide or symptoms that interfere with your ability to function. See your physician or mental health care professional promptly and get the help you deserve.

Dysthymia, a long-lasting but mild depression, can be even

harder to diagnose than major depression. Many mothers of young children find it hard to differentiate between dysthmia and the normal fatigue and stress of motherhood. If your baby is at least two years old and you've had mood issues for most of that time or longer, you may have this disorder.

The criteria for dysthymic disorder are a depressed mood for most of the day, more days than not, for at least two years, plus the presence of two or more of the following symptoms—provided that they are not due to substance abuse or a medical condition—to the degree that they cause distress or impairment in social, occupational, or other important functions:

- Poor appetite or overeating

- Insomnia or hypersomnia

- Low energy or fatigue

- Low self-esteem

- Poor concentration or difficulty making decisions

- Feelings of hopelessness

Again, *do not try to diagnose yourself based on these symptoms.* See a mental health care professional for a proper diagnosis and treatment.

Once a diagnosis of postpartum depression is made by a professional, treatment usually consists of a combination of medication and therapy. There is no shame in this treatment and it is not a sign of a flawed or weak character. Getting help is the mature and courageous response. Treatment will enable you to be the best mother you can be and to enjoy your family and your life.

In addition to therapy and appropriate medication, there are many self-help strategies that can alleviate postpartum depression, including a healthful diet, physical exercise, and relaxation practices. Many of these are included in the Get Your Body Back Program.

If you have symptoms of a postpartum mood disorder, it is important to see a mental health professional *before* you attempt to start the program. If you are in the throes of depression, it will be difficult, if not impossible, to find the resolve and focus needed for the program. Medication to address serotonin deficiency or other biochemical imbalances, along with counseling, may be necessary before you're in a frame of mind to stay motivated.

Once you are past the crisis point, the information and activities presented in these pages will be a wonderful adjunct to therapy and medication. The program will start you on an eating and exercise regime that can facilitate your recovery. In addition, these healthy habits will help you remain emotionally resilient and discourage recurrences of depression.

THE THYROID CONNECTION

One of the hidden reasons for depression, fatigue, and difficulty losing weight after childbirth is thyroid imbalance. Researchers have found that as many as 10 percent of postpartum women have autoimmune-related thyroid disorders.

The thyroid gland is a butterfly-shaped, walnut-size gland at the lower front of the neck. The gland produces thyroid hormones which circulate throughout the bloodstream and enter each cell. These hormones regulate cell temperature, cell function, and cell growth. In essence, every cell in the body requires thyroid hormone to function well. In the cells, a complex protein molecule binds to

DNA in a different way than it would without the presence of thyroid hormone. The production of thyroid hormone is controlled by brain signals to the pituitary gland, through the chemical TSH (thyroid simulating hormone).

There can be two main problems with thyroid function: low thyroid (hypothyroidism) and overactive thyroid (hyperthroidism). Hashimoto's thyroiditis is a prevalent autoimmune disorder that results in hypothyroidism. Graves disease is an autoimmune disorder that causes 70 percent of hyperthyroid cases. Both of these disorders involve a complex reaction of the immune system to the thyroid gland and a resulting imbalance. Genetics are thought to account for about half the predisposition to these problems. Other influences are the environment, infections, stress, and fluctuations of sex hormones (estrogen and progesterone).

In addition to a host of physical symptoms, thyroid imbalances can have mental effects. Hypothyroidism can cause depression, mental sluggishness, increased sleepiness, forgetfulness, difficulty concentrating, irritability, and emotional instability. People with hypothyroidism often complain of feeling exhausted and overwhelmed. Since these feelings are experienced by many mothers, thyroid issues are often overlooked.

On the hyperthyroid side of the spectrum, symptoms include anxiety, panic attacks, irritability, emotional swings, paranoia, aggression, and depression. Untreated hyperthyroid patients sometimes show signs of false elation, which is actually mania, resulting in poor judgment and abnormal behavior.

In general, hyperthyroidism tends to occur before the first two to three months after delivery have passed. Hypothyroidism usually occurs later, about four months after childbirth. These conditions may be transient, lasting a few months, or may develop into chronic problems.

The mental and physical symptoms of thyroid disease are easily confused with other problems, undiagnosed, or misdiagnosed. Self-diagnosis of a thyroid imbalance is virtually impossible, particularly when you're in the postpartum period, during which mood fluctuations can have so many origins.

For this reason, if you have postpartum mood disorder (or persistent physical symptoms) it is important to *have your thyroid tested*. Without taking the thyroid into account, treatments such as antidepressants and therapy may be only partially successful. You'll also be fighting an uphill battle to lose weight if you're hypothyroid.

Be aware that you may have to specifically request a full thyroid panel blood test, which includes measurement of T3 and T4, and TSH (the pituitary hormone, which controls functioning of the thyroid gland). Some physicians test T4 and T3 levels without obtaining a TSH measurement, an oversight that can lead to misdiagnosis.

If low thyroid is diagnosed, your physician will probably prescribe a synthetic thyroid hormone to be taken daily. With the correct dosage, these medications have virtually no side effects. Hyperthyroidism is treated with antithyroid drugs that sometimes have minor side effects. Blood tests will be required periodically to monitor dosages. Nursing mothers should consult with their physicians about the safety of these (and all) medications during lactation.

It should be fine to start the program in this book once your thyroid function is stabilized, but check with your physician first. Having a well-balanced thyroid will set the stage for success with the program. It will decrease your predisposition to emotional eating, get your metabolism on course, and give you the energy you need to be a healthy mom.

COMFORT FOODS AND EMOTIONAL EATING

Susan nibbles on chocolate throughout the day. She's stuck at home with two kids under the age of three and thinks she deserves a treat. She doesn't realize that the fluctuations in her blood sugar level are making her job as a mother even more tiring. The refined sugar is absorbed into her bloodstream and cells so rapidly that it is quickly depleted. This results in a letdown in her mood and energy level.

Before having a baby, Amy used to ignore the doughnut cart that made the office rounds twice a day. But now she always craves a pick-me-up. She's tired from interrupted sleep. She misses her baby. So she downs doughnuts and coffee to adjust her mood.

Leslie's eighteen-month-old baby is a fussy eater and mealtimes are frustrating. So Leslie shovels down the leftovers. Little dishes of pasta and pudding that are meant to fatten up the baby fatten up Mommy instead.

Joanne eats tortilla chips and salsa every day around six. By that time she's hungry for dinner, but wants to wait until her husband gets home. The baby gets cranky, and crunching on chips is an irresistible impulse.

Women with young children eat for many reasons besides hunger. Fatigue, anxiety, irritation, boredom, frustration, or cabin fever from long days at home. Feeling empty when we're at work and separated from the baby. Making up for other pleasures that we miss, such as sex, travel, partying, movies, or sleeping past the crack of dawn.

All too often, we use food in a misguided attempt to self-medicate. We turn to caffeine and sugar when we're tired and seeking energy. Pasta and potatoes when we want to calm down. Chips when we need to vent frustration. Creamy foods for comfort. The variations of emotional eating are endless.

Consider for a moment what you eat, when, and why. How often are you actually hungry and in need of nourishment? Probably when you first wake up. Perhaps at lunchtime, if you haven't eaten all morning. Maybe at dinnertime, if you wait too late to eat. But what about all the times in between?

It can be illuminating to keep a piece of paper in the kitchen for a few days to track what you eat, when, and how you're feeling at the time. Here's how my eating record looked on a day when I was home with baby Belinda:

Eating Record

TIME	WHAT	WHY
7 A.M.	Cereal and milk, coffee	Hungry
9 A.M.	Bagel and butter	Went in to the kitchen to get Belinda's formula, saw the bagel and it looked tasty. I'm already tired (up since 5:30) and need a break.
11 A.M	Cheese	Opened the fridge to get Belinda juice and had a craving to put something in my mouth.
1 P.M.	Soup, then cookies and coffee	I was a little hungry and soup seemed a sensible lunch. Then I was exhausted and needed coffee. Wanted something sweet to go with the coffee.

TIME	WHAT	WHY
3 P.M.	¾ dish of ice cream	Bought ice cream for Belinda when we went on our walk. She ate a little, then lost interest. I couldn't resist.
6 P.M.	Most of a yogurt; half a baby-food pasta	Belinda doesn't eat much, although she's a healthy weight. I'm frustrated and hungry so I polish off her food.
9 P.M.	Chicken, baked potato, and vegetable	Waited until Belinda was in bed and house was tidied to sit down and have dinner with Jonathan. I'd already eaten a dinner's worth of baby food at 6, but I wanted to have an adult meal and conversation.

If you read this record, you'll notice that I was actually hungry only once or twice during the day. But I had a lot of other reasons to eat!

Emotional eating is the number-one reason why diets fail. You know what's healthy, low-fat, etc. But somewhere in the deep recesses of your mind, countercravings speak louder than intellectual knowledge. You reach for a food that spoils your diet, even when you know better.

You succumb because you're trying to adjust a mood that's uncomfortable. It's habit. It's upbringing. Other people offer you food. A commercial on TV sparks a craving or you see a tempting food in the fridge. There are many triggers throughout the day. It's human to succumb. Forget about feeling guilty. But consider a better way.

The Get Your Body Back Program helps you overcome ingrained eating habits that are based on emotion instead of reason. Each part of the program deals with emotional eating in a specific way:

1. HELP for Moms provides a balance of foods that will supply you with a steady stream of energy. With moderate portions and frequent meals, you won't experience the highs and lows of blood sugar fluctuations. Since you won't be lacking nutrients, you'll be less vulnerable to filling yourself with food you don't need.

2. The Workable Workouts will make you more energetic and less prone to fatigue. Exercising will elevate your mood far longer than any candy bar can. It will reduce your stress load and give you confidence to meet the challenges of being a modern mom.

3. Mommy Care will provide ways to treat yourself without any backlash or guilt. True, your life is no longer your own. But there are still small indulgences outside the kitchen that you can enjoy.

Easy Alternatives to Comfort Foods

TRADITIONAL COMFORT FOOD	ALTERNATIVE
Ice cream and puddings	Low-fat yogurt
Candy, cake, and cookies	Fruit
Potato chips and tortilla chips	Apple chips, pretzels, air-popped popcorn

TRADITIONAL COMFORT FOOD	ALTERNATIVE
Heaping plate of pasta	Small (½–1 cup) portion of pasta
Bagels and rolls	Whole grain bread
Mashed potatoes	Baked potato with just a touch of butter
Beer and wine	Flavored seltzers

EATING FOR ENERGY

The common condition of anyone who has a baby under six months is fatigue. It's natural to turn to food for energy. The problem is that so many of the foods we reach for when we're tired actually *deplete* energy.

The secret of sustained energy is to eat small portions, frequent meals, and a balance of healthy foods. Drinking lots of water also elevates your energy level. The HELP for Moms Menu meets all these energy goals:

- Small portions of high-protein foods (eggs, meat, fish, non-fat dairy products)

- Small portions of complex carbohydrates (whole wheat breads, whole wheat or grain cereals, potatoes)

- Adequate fruits and vegetables to supply vitamins and minerals

- An emphasis on low-fat foods

- Plenty of water

Eating for Energy

ENERGY DRAINERS	ENERGY ADDERS
Candy	Apples, bananas, pears
Cookies, cakes, pastries	Citrus fruits
Sugary sodas	Flavored seltzer
Sugary cereals	Whole grain and wheat cereals
Too-large portions of starches	Small portions of pasta, potatoes, grains
Fatty and fried foods	Lean fish and poultry
"Junk food" snacks	Rice cakes, crackers, popcorn

THE SEROTONIN STORY

Serotonin is a neurochemical that functions in part as a neurotransmitter; it conveys messages from cell to cell throughout the nervous system. It has a profound impact on the brain and influences aspects of physiology such as body temperature, blood pressure, blood clotting, immunity, pain, digestion, sleep, and circadian (cyclical) body rhythms.

Serotonin dysfunction and imbalances are often associated with depression and anxiety. Serotonin problems are also indicated in extreme irritability, aggression, impulsivity, substance abuse, overeating, and bingeing. Some researchers have suggested that serotonin is a "surrogate parent" that discourages the wrong behavior, comforts us, and even helps us eat and sleep properly.

Serotonin imbalances can be the result of genetic predisposition, physical or emotional stress, and other factors. Giving birth creates a temporary hormone imbalance that includes a decline in serotonin levels. For some women this low serotonin state persists. Symptoms of low serotonin can include depression, fatigue, insomnia, pessimism, and diminished energy.

Serotonin has an important role in postpartum fitness because of the interplay between emotions and actions. A woman who is suffering from low-serotonin-related mood problems will find it difficult to stay with a healthy diet and exercise regularly. Many women overeat the wrong foods in an attempt to jump-start their serotonin function.

Low serotonin can influence food cravings and eating habits, although the pattern varies. In cases of major depression, people sometimes lose their appetite as their ability to take pleasure in food declines. But more frequently, women *over*eat to compensate for depleted serotonin and the resultant mood problems.

There is nothing inherently wrong with supplying your brain with additional serotonin by consuming carbohydrates. The problem lies in the type of carbohydrates that we choose and the size of the portions. Before food can spark serotonin production, it must make its way through the digestive system, a process that takes thirty to forty minutes. So we may keep eating and eating, seeking solace, without giving the digestive system enough time to respond. This is especially true for the rushed, distracted mom who eats standing up, hurrying to fill herself up before the baby cries.

It's clear that there is a biochemical basis for the phenomenon of "comfort foods" and bingeing when you're under stress. But what can you do to control the cravings?

The answer lies in keeping yourself supplied with a steady stream of the proper nutrients. The goal is to keep the serotonin from becoming depleted, so that stress-related food cravings don't occur. This is achieved by eating small, frequent meals that include low-fat complex carbohydrates; doing exercise and relaxation practices on a regular basis; plus communicating and connecting with the people you love as much as possible.

There are two types of carbohydrates: Simple and complex. Simple carbohydrates are sugars, such as glucose and fructose. Complex carbohydrates are starches, and include valuable sources of nutrition such as potatoes, rice, pasta, and whole grain or whole wheat bread.

While your instincts or habits may trick you into craving foods with high sugar content, these have little value in producing serotonin, and have a roller-coaster effect on blood sugar levels that, in turn, can exacerbate mood and energy problems. So it's wiser to choose from the list of complex carbohydrates. These foods can raise your serotonin level without undermining your weight loss goal—provided that you eat moderate portions and are careful of your sauces and condiments.

Some serotonin-boosting complex carbohydrates are:

- Whole wheat or whole grain bread

- Pasta

- White or brown rice

- Beans, peas, lentils

- Corn

- Potatoes

- Cooked cereal: wheat, rice, or oatmeal

- Whole grain cold cereal: shredded wheat, bran, corn-flakes.

These foods have several bonuses for new mothers. They're easy to prepare, simple, and satisfying. Serotonin-boosting foods supply energy to power muscles, which you'll need to carry and care for your ever-growing baby. They help to alleviate constipation, which is often a problem for many months after delivery. They're low-cost, and they taste delicious!

In addition to the serotonin-elevating foods, you need a diet that includes plenty of fresh fruits, vegetables, and complete proteins to fortify yourself against emotional upheaval. Water is also important, since dehydration can contribute to a feeling of mental confusion and stress.

If you suffer from depression, anxiety, or other diagnosed mood disorder, you may require a period of medication to restore your level of serotonin to proper functioning. Your doctor will most likely prescribe one of the SSRI family of medications such as Prozac, Zoloft, or Paxil.

The Get Your Body Back Program can be a valuable adjunct to a course of medication and therapy. The activities and menu enhance serotonin balance by giving you:

- A well-balanced diet containing lots of complex carbohydrates

- Smaller, more frequent meals

- Exercise, especially rhythmic exercise such as fitness walking

- Relaxation techniques.

EXERCISE TO ELEVATE YOUR MOOD

The baby has been fussy all morning. Now she's finally fallen asleep and looks like a perfect angel, snuggled in her crib. It's your first free moment since 6 A.M. and your instinct is to head to the kitchen to polish off last night's cake.

But wait. How long will that lift last? What about the letdown after the sugar rush? And the guilt! Here's another idea. Get out an exercise videotape and do a workout. Or put on your favorite music and dance around your living room for twenty minutes. Step onto your front lawn to stretch in the sun (as long as you can still hear the baby if she wakes up, of course). These antidotes to stress and fatigue will give you the up without the down.

Here's another common scenario: You're at work and it's lunchtime. You're exhausted from having been up with the baby twice last night. Nonetheless, you miss him and feel sad that you're separated all day. You're not looking forward to the same old lunch routine: a crowded diner, a lunch laden with extra calories, a rush to finish and get back to work. You know that after you eat you'll be in for the afternoon slump.

How about a change in the routine? Can you dash out to a gym or studio for an exercise class? Or take a brisk walk for a half hour, then eat a light salad? You'll be sharper at your afternoon tasks, and more energized to enjoy your time with the baby when you get home.

Exercise is a wonderful paradox—both relaxing and energetic at the same time. It is a tranquilizer and a stimulant. Exercise gives you the psychological relief you seek without the worthless fat and sugar of junk food or sweets. There's no downside, no slump after the indulgence. No side effects, no guilt, no ambivalence.

After you exercise, your body may feel slightly tired for a brief time. But your mind will be refreshed. You'll feel more awake, energetic, optimistic. Better able to concentrate on intellectual tasks and work. Readier to respond cheerfully to your baby's needs. Exercise will give you the stamina to keep up with the demands of motherhood, and the confidence that you can do it.

It's always been known that walking, stretching, dancing, swimming, and other forms of physical activity can clear the mind, lift the spirits, and increase energy. Now researchers have uncovered a number of physiological reasons for this common knowledge.

First, sustained exercise can raise serotonin levels. One study found that steady exercise increased not only serotonin production, but also serotonin activity, even for several weeks after training stopped. Exercise also stimulates the production of endorphins, the neurotransmitters that can induce feelings of joy, well-being, and euphoria.

Researchers are finding that exercise can both alleviate and prevent incidences of depression. A study of twelve people with moderate or severe depression found that their symptoms were reduced by 30 to 50 percent after only ten days of walking on a treadmill for thirty minutes a day. This is even faster relief than afforded by antidepressants, which generally take two to four weeks to take effect. This research indicates that if you walk your baby (briskly) in the stroller for a half hour a day, it should lift your mood.

The surest way to enhance your mood is to do at least thirty minutes of exercise. But something is always better than nothing. Five minutes of stretching, ten minutes of fast walking, or whatever you can manage will help your mood.

If you are a working mother, fitting exercise into your busy schedule is a good investment. During aerobic exercise, blood flow to the brain increases. Studies have shown that this can improve memory, concentration, verbal fluency, and creative problem-solving ability. Women often feel a diminishment of these skills during the first year after childbirth. If you have difficulty concentrating on work—whether it's because of interrupted sleep, hormonal fluctuations, or a preoccupation with your baby—a workout can sharpen your mental processes.

ALL MOMS ARE WORKING

I've always thought that it's unfair to reserve the term "working mothers" for women who work at a paying job. *All* mothers of young children work hard, one way or another. And we're all vulnerable to different types of stress and emotional eating.

If you're staying at home to care for your baby full-time, you probably feel secure that you're doing the right thing for the little one. But you may have money worries. Regrets about giving up your job. Concerns about getting your career back on track once you return to the workforce. You may feel bored and isolated or miss intellectual challenge and adult company. So you snack throughout the day to relieve boredom and frustration.

If you work outside the home, you may struggle with ambivalence and guilt about leaving your baby. You're stressed by your dual roles. You're not sure if it's best for your baby to be spending so much time away from you. You worry about the quality of your childcare. You miss your baby and feel pangs throughout the day. You turn to indulgent lunches and snacks for comfort.

If you try to pursue a career at home when you have a baby (as I did), it's hard to concentrate. You constantly feel distracted and caught between two roles. Even when you have a sitter watching the baby while you work, you're tempted to respond to every cry you can't help overhearing.

One advantage that women who work outside the home have is in the weight-loss department. Research has found that women who return to work earlier after having a baby lose more weight and lose it faster than women who stay at home. This is hardly surprising. When you're home with the baby, you're home with food. You have endless opportunities to visit the fridge and pantry. In fact, it's impossible to stay out of the kitchen, since you're always running in for a bottle or for a baby food feeding session.

If you're a home-based worker, there are great advantages: You don't waste time commuting, you can be nearer to your beloved baby, you don't have to spend money on clothes, transportation, etc. The disadvantage is the proximity to food. In general, home-based workers are prone to gaining weight.

How to Control Emotional Eating

If you're a full-time homemaker:

- Seek professional help if you have postpartum depression or a mood disorder.

- Purge your house of the comfort foods that sabotage your diet.

- Set structured meal and snack times for yourself.

- Every time you find yourself reaching for an unscheduled snack, have a glass of water instead.

- Be sure to socialize with other new moms. Join or form playgroups so you have a schedule.

- Be outside with your baby as much as possible; it's good for both your moods.

- Exercise every day you can . . . your baby will enjoy the routine of a daily walk.

If you have a home-based business:

- Seek professional help if you have postpartum depression or a mood disorder.

- Purge your house of overly tempting diet-sabotagers.

- Establish meal and snack times for yourself; stay out of the kitchen the rest of the day.

- Keep a frequently refilled water bottle in your home office. Every time you feel like an unscheduled snack, drink water instead.

- If you get too stressed out, take advantage of your freedom. Put on a workout videotape, go for a walk, or just go outside to stretch and breathe.

- Get dressed for work in fitted clothes. If you stay in loose, schlumpy clothing all day, you'll feel less motivated to get fit.

If you work outside the home:

- Seek professional help if you have postpartum depression or a mood disorder.

- Pack healthy snacks and lunches from the HELP for Moms Menus.

- Limit social lunches to once or twice a week so you're not too tempted by what others are eating.

- Establish snack times for yourself.

- Keep a frequently refilled water bottle by your desk. Every time you feel like an unscheduled snack, drink water instead.

- Try to exercise during your lunch hour two or three times a week.

- Pop your baby in the stroller for a fitness walk as soon as you get home, when the weather allows.

CHAPTER 3

THE HEALTHY EATING LIGHT PLAN (**HELP**) FOR MOMS

The Healthy Eating Light Plan (HELP) for Moms is based on the time-tested, proven principles of nutrition for safe, gradual weight loss. This eating plan does not claim to be groundbreaking or guarantee that you'll lose an incredible amount of weight in record time. Instead, it's a moderately paced way to lose extra weight while enhancing your health and energy.

Right now, you have a tremendous responsibility to your baby to stay even-keeled and strong. It's the wrong time to experiment with a radical diet. Also, you probably don't have the inclination to work out complicated food combinations and calculations when so much of your thought process is focused on the baby. After following this plan for a few months, you can expect to kiss your baby fat good-bye!

TWO BASIC APPROACHES

1. **Follow the monthly meal plans.** Each month of the program gives seven days of plans for five meals: breakfast, midmorning mini-meal, lunch, midafternoon mini-meal, and dinner. If you want to keep it very, very simple, just follow these meal plans for each day of the week. Then repeat the menu for the following weeks of that month. You'll find that the routine of repeating meal plans makes the program practical and easy. If

you are nursing, select the appropriate amount of breast-feeding bonus foods to supply additional nutrition. *Or:*

2. **Design your own meal options.** If you want more flexibility, you can substitute various lunches, dinners, and mini-meals from different days. You can also use this method to avoid any foods that don't appeal to you. If you don't like fish, pick a meat dinner from another day. If you don't touch red meat, choose a pasta or poultry entree. If you don't feel like having hot soup for lunch, have a sandwich or salad. You can mix and match occasionally without sabotaging your weight loss efforts. However, if you're breast-feeding, the best way to ensure maximum nutritional value is to stay with the meal plans most days.

THE HELP RULES FOR WEIGHT LOSS

In addition to following the meal plans, a major goal of the program is to understand and follow the four basic rules for healthy eating when trying to lose weight. Hopefully, after three months these rules will become second nature. Then when you're ready to return to more flexible eating, you can continue to stay in good shape.

RULE #1: EAT EARLY

Nocturnal eating sabotages many women who carefully control their food intake throughout the day. It's not just *what* you eat, it's *when* you eat it. About twelve hours after you wake up, your metabolism slows down dramatically. The sun sets on your calorie-burning ability and whatever you eat is more likely to be stored as fat.

Your metabolism is fastest in the morning and afternoon, slows down in the evening, and descends to its lowest level at night. As metabolism slows, the fat cells take up the slack by storing calories. Your body needs fewer calories to function and the overload is stored as fat.

To lose weight at a healthy rate while still consuming enough nutrients, it's imperative to eat your dinner as early as possible, then close the kitchen door. Try to finish dinner by 6:30 P.M. If you're nursing, have one bonus food at 8:00 in the evening. If you absolutely know that you won't be able to survive without a snack, save your dessert and have it at 8. Otherwise, drink lots of water all evening and stay out of the kitchen as much as possible after dinner.

There are certainly drawbacks to eating early and it can be a sacrifice—but a worthwhile one. If you stick to early eating, you'll see faster weight-loss results.

One problem is that if you eat dinner when your baby is awake, you may not be able to have an uninterrupted meal. This makes dining less relaxing. On the other hand, you're less likely to overeat.

Another issue is that your husband may not be back from work early enough to join you in an early dinner. For a while, you may have to miss the pleasure of sitting down and eating together as adults. If this is your situation, designate one night a week as a "dinner date," when you eat together at a later hour, after baby is in bed. But on the ordinary evenings, eat early. It will have a tremendous effect on the success of your weight loss efforts.

MOTHER'S HELPER HINT: If you want to prepare dinner for a partner who comes home later, buy a supply of microwavable segmented dinner plates with covers. Cook the meal early and eat your portion early. Save his portion in the plate so that all he has to do is pop it into the microwave later to heat it up—while you stay out of the kitchen to avoid temptation.

RULE #2: EAT LESS, BUT MORE FREQUENTLY

Tara's friends affectionately call her an earth mother. She carries her baby against her breast in a Snugli as she bakes her own bread. A vegetarian, she cooks delicious dishes brimming with organic goodness. Refined sugar and junk food never pass her lips. But despite the healthfulness of her diet, she's still carrying around 20 extra pounds six months after having her baby. Although she's nursing full-time, the weight is not coming off.

Tara's problem lies in portion size. Even the healthiest complex carbohydrates can be fattening if the portions are too large. This leads to a lot of confusion about dieting. Is it inevitably fattening to eat pasta, bread, grains, potatoes, and dairy products? The answer is no . . . but a qualified no. You are welcome to partake of these foods, but you have to be careful of portion size.

The meal plans in this program provide portions that supply ample nutrition, without excess calories that will be stored in fat cells. These portions won't leave you hungry, but they're probably smaller than what you're used to seeing on your plate. However, there is a positive side to this sacrifice. Although portions are smaller, you can also eat more frequently. The idea is to turn you into one of those "naturally thin" people, who are accustomed to eating modest portions.

Jessica returned to her prepregnancy weight and shape three months after delivering a gorgeous 10-pound baby boy. She claims that she doesn't know how she lost the 35 pounds she gained during pregnancy so fast, because she "eats all day long." But if you have lunch with Jessica, you'll find that she eats slowly and is satisfied with small portions.

There are a few young mothers who can consume huge portions of food frequently throughout the day and still stay slim. But they are rare, and usually under thirty. Most women who remain naturally slim have a natural inclination to consume small meals. The rest of us have to work hard at developing this habit.

What if you prefer to eat two or three big meals, instead of three modest meals and two snacks each day? Sorry, but it won't work. For the three months of the program, you'll have to make an adjustment if you want to see results.

If you eat all your calories in two large meals, you're taking in more than your body can utilize at one time. The excess will be stored in your fat cells. The long gaps between eating can cause fluctuations in your mood and energy level, and slow your metabolism. You might feel virtuous because you're only eating twice a day, but it's doubtful that you'll lose weight.

If you consume all your calories in three meals a day, you're probably still taking in a little more than you can utilize at each meal. Your weight will plateau or creep up steadily over the years, and with each ensuing pregnancy.

If you divide your calories into five portions a day, however, your body will be able to utilize these calories more effectively. You'll have little excess to store as fat. Your energy level will stay steady. Your mood will stabilize and you'll have more patience with your baby, your spouse, your co-workers. You may be hungry when you wake up in the morning, but you won't feel deprived during the day, since you'll be eating every three hours.

Women who want to lose weight sometimes make the mistake of starving themselves for half the day, waiting for lunchtime or even dinner before they allow a morsel to pass their lips. This is one of the most destructive diet mistakes you can make. And if you have the responsibility of taking care of a young baby, it's not even an option.

When you're not getting enough nourishment, your body starts to break down muscle to feed itself, leaving you weakened.

You are prone to depression, anxiety, and irritability. Your metabolism slows down. Whatever weight you shed is likely to come back as soon as you start eating normally. Drastic dieting also puts stress on your internal organs and can weaken your immune system.

What time you consume your five meals depends on your schedule. The pattern is to eat within a half hour of rising, so you don't start the day hungry, then eat every two and a half to three hours. If your baby wakes up at dawn, here's how it might look:

Breakfast: 6:30 A.M.

Mini-Meal: 9:30 A.M.

Lunch: 12:30 P.M.

Mini-Meal: 3:30 P.M.

Dinner: 6:00 P.M.

Bonus food if nursing and/or dessert saved from dinner (optional): 8:00 P.M.

NOTE: *Nursing moms can add one or more additional bonus foods at the time of their choice.*

Eating five times a day ensures that you never go hungry. But you can't consume five huge meals a day and expect to lose weight. Portion control and choosing high-value foods is the key.

We can all learn from certain preschoolers, when it comes to portion size and eating patterns. My three-year-old, Belinda, eats very small portions at mealtimes. And every few hours she requests a cup of milk or a snack. Although my instinct as a mother is to wish she'd finish a heaping plate of food at dinner, she's always been a perfect size. She has boundless energy for running, jumping, playing, dancing, and giggling. Clearly, her own little internal wisdom is telling her how to get nourishment.

One of the big bonuses of eating small, more frequent meals is the energy surplus. How do you feel after Thanksgiving dinner or a lengthy meal in an Italian restaurant? Satiated, perhaps, but also sleepy. This is fine once in a while, during a holiday or after a special night out. But you can't afford the energy drain on an average day, when you're taking care of a baby, perhaps working at an outside job, running a household. You need all the steady strength you can muster.

Eating smaller, more frequent meals also affords an advantage to career-oriented moms. When you eat a heavy meal, your stomach diverts blood supply away from your brain. This contributes to a feeling of mental sluggishness. Light meals give you the fuel without the brain drain. The result is more mental acuity and better concentration.

Eating small, more frequent meals also supplies a more stable level of blood sugar. This helps you manage stress, control your emotions, and maintain calm in the face of chaos. You have more resilience to cope with all the demands of your day. It's both calming and stimulating at the same time—just what all mommies need.

RULE #3: EAT LOW-FAT FOODS

High-fat foods are already in a handy form for fat storage. Fat cells can scoop them right up and store them as fat, frustrating your attempts at dieting. Carbohydrates and proteins require more effort to be converted into fat. So while overeating any food will put on extra weight, high-fat foods will weigh you down the most.

High-fat foods are also the least efficient sources of energy. Carbohydrates are the best source of energy for organs and cells.

Protein is optimal for concentration and muscle growth. Fat is only good for storing fat.

Some people are born with a greater and larger number of fat cells than other individuals, a genetically determined factor that you can't control. Naturally svelte women have smaller and fewer fat cells than those with a propensity toward obesity, but this is only part of the picture. The other factor stems from what you eat. Fat cells are alive. When you eat more than you can metabolize, especially high-fat foods, your fat cells get bigger. When you reduce fat intake, your fat cells shrink.

You can't kill off fat cells and you wouldn't want to. You have to give these fat cells some credit because for most of womankind's history they've served an important function. The purpose of fat cells is to store calories you don't immediately require, and release them when needed. As a woman, you're preprogrammed to store fat for lean times, to protect your offspring during pregnancy and lactation.

Diets with severe caloric restrictions can actually make your fat cells *more* efficient at storing fat. When you're not getting enough food, fat-storing lipogenic enzymes become activated and multiply. This enables your body to be more effective at storing fat after the diet (or famine) ends. It's a survival mechanism. You can't click it off just because we live in the land of plenty. Your fat cells don't know if you're starving because you want to look like a model or because the crops failed.

That's why the HELP for Moms Menu emphasizes small, frequent, nourishing meals instead of starvation tactics. We never want to switch those fat cells into starvation survival mode. We want to encourage moderately paced, permanent loss of extra fat and cultivate a taste for low-fat food choices.

There are many reasons beyond getting back to your prepregnancy weight to permanently adopt a diet lower in fat. Excess fat is linked to hypertension, high cholesterol, risk of heart disease, and other ills. While these ailments may seem like remote possibilities now, by the time your baby is grown up, you may be at risk. A low-fat diet will help you stay healthy so you can enjoy your grandchildren as well as your children!

One complaint that many people have about low-fat food is flavor. It's true that high-fat foods can be absolutely delicious, sensuous, and seductive. But low-fat food doesn't have to taste like cardboard. You can make low-fat meals look, smell, and taste enticing with the creative use of herbs, spices, and fresh ingredients.

RULE #4: DRINK LOTS OF WATER

Water curbs your appetite, breaks down fat, flushes out toxins, and performs a host of other miracles. How much is enough? You'll need to let your own body tell you. Generally, eight 8-ounce glasses a day for nonnursing women and ten 8-ounce glasses for lactating women is quite sufficient.

When you're drinking a great deal of water, you want to be sure that it's as pure and safe as possible. Although tap water is safe in most communities, it's a good idea to do some research. Check with your local health department, a consumer advocacy group, or the Environmental Protection Agency (EPA) to find out about your local water supply. Inquire if there are high levels of chemicals from possible seepage or run-off from farms or industry. Find out if there is leaching of lead or other metals from pipes. You can even have a laboratory do a water analysis if you're concerned. And you may have to look into the possibility of having your plumbing pipes replaced if there is leaching from lead solder.

If you're not sure about your tap water, you can buy bottled water, although it becomes cumbersome and expensive to haul those heavy jugs home. You'll need 3½ to 4½ gallons each week.

Also, even some bottled brands have high chemical, metal, or salt levels. A better option is to install a high-quality filter on your kitchen tap so that all the water for cooking and drinking is filtered.

OTHER BEVERAGES. Even a new mom cannot live by water alone. Here are suggested guidelines for other beverages that you may want to have occasionally, *in addition* to your 8–10 glasses of water:

- *Plain or flavored seltzers:* One or two a day, if you choose.

- *Milk:* Select nonfat (skim) milk or 1 percent low-fat milk when it's part of the menu.

- *Fruit juice:* Drink only pure fruit juice that has no fructose or other additives. Have no more than one 6-ounce cup a day diluted with a little water.

- *Coffee:* Limit your intake to no more than two cups per day. Use a small amount of nonfat milk if desired. If you want a sweetener, use no more than a teaspoon of sugar; avoid artificial sweeteners.

- *Tea:* No more than two cups of caffeinated tea, with a dash of nonfat milk and sugar if desired. Herbal tea, hot or cold, is a good choice to provide a change of taste without caffeine or calories. However, if you're breast-feeding, be careful of the type of herbs the tea contains. Safe choices include rose hip teas and noncaffeinated teas flavored with fruit such as orange, raspberry, or lemon.

- *Beer, Wine, and Alcohol:* Alas, alcoholic drinks do contain empty calories. So during the three months of the program, limit yourself to a few drinks a *week* (not a day). Choose light beer instead of regular beer. If you have a cocktail, mix the alcohol with seltzer and just a splash of juice.

- *Regular sodas:* None. They are loaded with sugar, caffeine, and nonnutritional calories.

- *Diet sodas:* Try to avoid diet drinks, especially if you're nursing. Artificial sweeteners and other chemicals in these sodas make them undesirable.

DIET DRUGS AND HERBS

If only there were a diet pill that worked without the risk of side effects . . . what an indulgent world it would be. But despite the relentless research of pharmaceutical companies, none exists. Every so often, a new diet drug emerges, hope blossoms, people lose weight, then gain it back, side effects arise, and so on.

Even the wisdom of thousands of years of herbal medicine has failed to find a secret of weight control. There are a number of herbal diet aids on the market. Some may have limited success for some people, if used in conjunction with diet and exercise. The tricky issue is that even these "natural" weight-loss pills can turn out to be unsafe for people with certain conditions.

Whether you're nursing or not, when you have a baby you're in a highly responsible position. This is not the time to be experimenting with diet pills or herbs that might cause physical or emotional side effects. You need to stay at the top of your game and be a little conservative. Get fit the tried-and-true, completely safe way: with a low-fat, high-nutrition diet and sensible exercise.

FROZEN FOODS

Fresh foods are always preferable to frozen from a nutritional standpoint. Try to buy fresh vegetables instead of frozen whenever possible. Fresh vegetables contain more "living" nutrition, and they have better flavor and color. Fresh fruit is also preferable, when it's available. When you select canned fruit, look for brands that are packaged in their own juices, without heavy syrup.

Meals cooked with fresh ingredients are more nutritious than frozen dinners, and also better tasting. However, in the real world, there may be times when you're too busy and/or tired to prepare even the simplest recipes. On these nights, you can heat up an extra portion of a meal from a previous night that you've frozen. Or you can opt to have a prepackaged frozen dinner as a meal substitute once or twice a week. You'll find a vast range of choices at most supermarkets, including many low-fat selections.

Look for frozen meals with these qualities:

- Less than 350 calories

- A low percentage of calories from fat

- Minimal preservatives and additives

- A good balance of protein and complex carbohydrates

THE FRESH FRUIT OPTION

Many women find that they don't feel satisfied unless they have something sweet for dessert, especially after dinner. To accommodate this taste, many of the meal plans offer a sweet treat for dessert: a few cookies, a diet brownie or pudding, or a serving of frozen yogurt. The calorie counts and other nutritional values for the day are calculated with this specific dessert.

However, if you feel satisfied with a piece of fruit after dinner, you're encouraged to substitute this healthy option. Any evening that you feel inclined, forego the suggested dessert and have the following instead:

- A whole apple, banana, pear, peach, or plum

- A whole orange, nectarine, or tangerine

- A quarter of a cantaloupe or a wedge of honeydew melon (7" × 2")

- A cup of blueberries, strawberries, cherries, or raspberries

Obviously, having fruit for dessert is more nutritious than a cookie, cake, or ice cream substitute. But if fruit leaves you craving more and you raid the cookie jar later that night, it's not going to do you much good. Try the fruit option a few nights and see if you can develop a taste for this healthy habit.

CHAPTER 4

THE BREAST-FEEDING BALANCE

Breast-feeding is widely acknowledged to be the best way to nourish a young baby. Breast milk supplies babies with food that is perfectly suited to their needs. No matter how advanced formulas become, they can never match or improve upon nature.

Nursing allows women to pass disease-fighting antibodies on to their babies. As a result, breast-fed babies generally make fewer trips to the pediatrician. Reports have shown that breast-feeding offers some protection against bronchitis, earache, pneumonia, and influenza. Breast-fed babies are less likely to develop asthma, diabetes, cancer, or obesity in childhood. They respond better to vaccines and their brains seem to develop faster. Breast-fed babies are three times less likely to be hospitalized than those who are bottle-fed.

Babies who are breast-fed have a lower incidence of digestive problems. A study of 600 mothers and babies from birth to age two found that children who were nursed for at least thirteen weeks had significantly less vomiting and diarrhea than formula-fed babies, even after nursing stopped.

Babies who are breast-fed also develop healthier teeth. They use more muscles to suck from the breast than from the bottle, which encourages the development of straighter teeth. They are less likely to develop cavities from milk, formula, or juice pooling around their developing teeth. And they are less prone to thumb-sucking habits.

Breast milk is satisfying to babies because it is rich in protein at the beginning of the nursing session, and contains more fat at the end to produce a feeling of fullness. Breast-feeding babies tend to eat just the right amount, since they suck until they are satisfied, instead of being encouraged to finish a whole bottle they really don't need. This can reduce the possibility of weight problems later in life for the child.

There is also a strong emotional reward involved in breast-feeding. Many mothers find nursing to be an incredibly fulfilling, magical experience. When else in your life can you provide a human being with complete emotional, nutritional, and physical satisfaction? When you're holding the baby to your breast, she has everything she needs in the world: ideal nourishment, the closeness of your arms, the smell and warmth of your body, the sight of your smile and shining eyes. No wonder it's so easy for babies to fall asleep blissfully at the end of a nursing session.

Breast-feeding has practical advantages, as well. You can save about $100 a month by not buying formula. You won't have to worry about purifying water, mixing, storing, sterilizing bottles, etc. Breast milk is the safest way to feed a young baby and, in many ways, the most convenient.

Yet despite all these advantages, the rate of breast-feeding is generally low in the United States. According to the Surgeon General, only 29 percent of new mothers breast-feed until their babies are six months old, a crucial period of development.

What are the reasons for this low rate, in a society where people are well educated and concerned about health? Sometimes mothers find nursing painful, uncomfortable, or inhibiting to their freedom. Occasionally babies do not flourish on breast milk, indicating a problem with milk production or an allergic response. There are rare cases where breast-feeding is counter indicated, such as when mothers are HIV-positive or infants have a metabolic disorder.

However, the most common reason for abandoning nursing is undoubtedly the pressure of working outside the home. Over half of American women with children under the age of one work outside the home. While it is certainly possible to breast-feed and work full-time—with dedication and a breast pump—it can be difficult and discouraging. Many women find that despite their best efforts, their milk supply dwindles once they return to work and rely on the pump.

BREAST-FEEDING AND YOUR BODY

It's clear that breast-feeding is good for your baby's body. There are also many physical benefits for you. Initially, breast-feeding helps your uterus contract, which encourages your abdomen to return to its normal shape. Lactation often stops menstruation for six to twelve months after childbirth (although this is not a reliable means of birth control). Your breasts will remain fuller than usual during lactation and you'll have that nursing mother's glow.

Breast-feeding can help your body conserve iron, if you suffered from iron-deficiency anemia during pregnancy. Some studies suggest that women who breast-feed have lower incidences of hip fractures, ovarian cancer, premenopausal breast cancer, and uterine cancer later in life.

Okay, now for the big question: Will breast-feeding help you lose weight? For a long time, nutritionists believed the answer was an unequivocal "Yes!" It was thought that nursing women could lose weight on 2700 calories per day, which is 500 calories above the Recommended Daily Allowance (RDA) of 2200 calories per day for adult women. I'm sorry to say that current thinking is more complicated.

First, the bad news. Research studies, as well as common experience, have found that many nursing mothers do not lose all their extra weight when they consume 2700 calories a day. Other studies have found nursing does not confer an automatic advantage when it comes to weight loss.

One study compared fifty-six new mothers, divided into groups who were nursing exclusively, not nursing, and mixing breast and bottle. Women were tracked after birth, at three and six months postpartum. The results found that there was no difference in the rate of weight loss between the three groups. However, the mothers who were feeding formula exclusively did consume fewer calories than the nursing moms, which may account for the results. It may signify that weight-loss comparisons level out because nursing mothers tend to eat more.

A large-scale study by the First European Congress on Obesity followed 1423 women for a year after giving birth. This study also found no significant weight-loss differences between nursing and nonnursing mothers.

However, this study and others have found that weight gain *during* pregnancy is the chief barometer of who loses and who does not. Women who gain more than the recommended amount during pregnancy have greater difficulty returning to prepregnancy weight. It's not surprising that the more you gain the more you have to take off.

Now for the good news: A study at the Children's Nutrition Research Center at Baylor College of Medicine in Texas found that women could successfully nurse their babies on far fewer than 2700 calories a day. The women in the study consumed an average of approximately 2186 calories a day, which fully nourished their babies while allowing the mothers to lose extra pounds slowly and steadily.

Of course, both your nutritional needs and your weight loss

will depend on whether or not you are nursing exclusively, mixing formula and/or food and breast milk, or just nursing once or twice a day. Your activity level, metabolism, genetics, and pregnancy weight gain are also important factors.

Your weight-loss potential varies during different periods of lactation. For the first four to six months of nursing (and during pregnancy), your pituitary gland produces high levels of a hormone called prolactin. This clever hormone is not only responsible for milk production, it also increases your appetite.

From a survival standpoint, it's smart for the same hormone that produces milk to encourage you to eat more. But it can make it difficult for you to control your portion sizes and craving for high-fat foods. So the extra calories you burn making breast milk may be counteracted by your desire (and need) to eat more.

But don't despair, there's good news. At four to six months postpartum, prolactin levels return to normal even if you're still breast-feeding. This makes it easier to stay with a diet and to reap the benefits of breast-feeding. It means that if you're sensible about eating and exercise, it can be quite beneficial to both your figure and your baby to keep nursing until baby's first birthday.

WHERE AND WHEN DOES THE WEIGHT GO?

Weight loss after childbirth is highly individual. But let's look at the experience of a theoretical "typical" woman who started off normal weight and gained 32 pounds during pregnancy:

Infant at birth:	8 pounds
Placenta:	1 pound
Amniotic fluid:	2 pounds
Weight loss after delivery:	11 pounds

Increased blood volume:	3 pounds
Enlarged uterus:	3 pounds
Extra fluid:	<u>3 pounds</u>
Weight loss in first few weeks:	9 pounds
Increase in breast tissue:	3 pounds
Increase in fat stores:	<u>9 pounds</u>
Weight that may require effort to lose:	12 pounds

In this example, the mother may find that the last 12 pounds do not melt away if she eats the same way she did before pregnancy. How difficult it will be to return to her postpartum weight will depend on her diet, activity level, genetics, and condition before pregnancy. If a woman starts from a normal or overweight condition, and gains more than 30 pounds during pregnancy, she will have additional fat stores to lose.

After the first few weeks, when does the remaining weight come off? This answer is also highly variable. One study reported that first-time mothers lose the most during the first trimester. Traditionally, however, the second postpartum trimester is considered to be the golden window of weight loss. By the sixth month, weight loss generally levels off unless a concentrated effort is made to diet and exercise.

Remember, it's not fair to judge your progress by the scale alone if you're breast-feeding (or even if you're not). Your breasts will weigh 2 to 3 pounds more than usual as long as you're nursing. Enjoy your voluptuous figure while it lasts and don't worry about the numbers. Your body will never be as beautiful and miraculous as it is while you're growing your baby with your milk.

EATING FOR TWO?

The Healthy Eating Light Plan depends on portion control, low-fat food choices, and the right balance of nutrition, rather than mere calorie counting. However, the inevitable question arises: How many more calories can I have if I'm breast-feeding?

To a large extent, this depends on how often you're nursing. There is a big difference between nursing "full-time" to provide a young baby with all the nutrition he needs and nursing once or twice a day for comfort and closeness. A common mistake a new mom makes is that she continues to "eat for two" when, in fact, her baby is getting most of his nutrition elsewhere and breast milk production is greatly diminished.

Here is an assessment that will help you categorize your breast-feeding status. See which category bests fits your pattern.

Breast-feeding Status

Full-timer:

- Your baby relies exclusively on breast milk, or

- Your baby eats a little food but drinks only breast milk instead of milk or formula.

- You have three or more nursing sessions a day.

- You are nursing to provide your baby's primary nourishment.

Part-timer:

- Your baby takes formula or milk in addition to breast milk.

- Your baby eats three meals a day of baby food or other solid food.

- You have two or fewer nursing sessions a day.

- You are nursing primarily for comfort, closeness, and some nutrition.

If you're a full-timer, you should consume 500 calories worth of the breast-feeding bonus foods listed below each day. If you're a part-timer, use your judgment and have between 150 and 500 calories worth of bonus foods, depending on how many times you nurse a day, how you feel, and how your baby is growing. You can have these bonus foods any time of the day, with a final bonus at 8 P.M. These bonus foods are especially selected to boost your calcium intake, as well as provide extra nutrition for you and your baby.

Breast-feeding Bonus Foods

Each day, select between 100 and 500 calories worth of these foods and beverages, depending on how often you are breast-feeding and how you feel.

Milk, 1%, 1 cup
   Look for organic milk while
   nursing.
	100 calories

Milkshake, banana
   1% milk, 1 cup
   1 medium banana
	220 calories

Soy beverage w/ added calcium,
   1 cup
   vanilla, almond, or
   plain flavor
	100–150 calories

Yogurt, 1 cup	120–240 calories
Select the flavor of your choice. Avoid products containing aspartame or other artificial sweeteners.	
Frozen yogurt, ½ cup	100–200 calories
Select the flavor of your choice. Avoid brands with artificial sweeteners or additives.	
Cheese, 1 ounce	80–110 calories
Cheddar, Colby, Gouda, or Edam	
Cottage cheese, 1 cup	180–220 calories
Low-fat plain or w/ pineapple	
Eggs, hard-boiled, 2 large	160 calories
Egg salad	210 calories
2 large eggs, hard-boiled, mashed with 1 tablespoon light mayonnaise and a dash of salt	
Eggs, scrambled	180 calories
2 large eggs, cooked w/ butter or canola spray	
Almonds, 1 ounce, blanched or raw	170 calories
Tofu, set with calcium, ½ cup	183 calories
Cereal, calcium-fortified, 1 cup	100–150 calories

Potato, baked, w/cheese   225 calories
   1 medium potato, baked
   in skin w/ 1 ounce cheddar
   cheese melted on top

NOTE ON DESSERTS: *If you're nursing, it's a good idea to substitute frozen yogurt, health food store cookies, or fruit for any of the "chocolatey" cookies, puddings, and pies on the Menu.*

The HELP for Moms Menu with full-timer bonus foods provides 2000–2100 calories a day, which should prove satisfying for you and your baby. The key is *quality*. Eating 2100 calories of a diet that includes high-fat and junk food could be inadequate nutritionally for nursing. But with the foods that are offered on the HELP for Moms meal plans—selected for their high nutritional value and balance—it should be sufficient.

Reducing the fat in your diet shouldn't have any effect on your baby's growth, and may even be a healthful influence. Some research has suggested that women who limit fat intake increase their milk production and produce milk that has a higher protein content. Of course, both your weight loss and your baby's weight gain should be supervised by a qualified doctor.

If you're providing all or most of your baby's nutrition (no milk or formula), you need to lose weight slowly, no more than one pound per week. Use common sense as your guide, and take in more food if you're feeling hungry or deprived.

Most importantly, you should be monitoring your baby's weight with your physician, to make sure the child is getting enough nourishment and gaining nicely. If baby's weight gain is slow, it may or may not be linked to your diet. There are many reasons for inadequate milk production and for babies to fail to gain weight. Seek advice for your particular situation from your doctor.

Most likely, however, you will find that the nutritional value of the HELP for Moms Menu with the added bonus foods will give you and your baby exactly what you need to thrive. You lose weight gradually and your baby gains steadily.

EATING FOR THREE AND OTHER CHALLENGES

Theoretically, if you're breast-feeding twins or triplets full-time, you need to increase your caloric intake by 500 calories for each additional child you're nursing. Realistically, however, nursing and caring for more than one infant is such a demanding job that you may want to wait until they're weaned before embarking on this book's weight-loss plan. Meanwhile, you can set the stage for fitness by going on walks with your double (or triple) stroller, drinking more water, and cutting down on fats and high-sugar foods.

If you have special health challenges while nursing, consult with your physician or a nutritionist to adapt the meal plan to your needs. These conditions include but are not limited to diabetes, high blood pressure, and iron-deficiency anemia.

GETTING ENOUGH FLUID

If you still feel hungry when following the meal plans and adding breast-feeding bonus foods, be sure that you're not actually starved for fluids. Nursing moms often mistake thirst for hunger.

Try to drink ten glasses of water a day. One way to remember is to drink a glass of water every time you give the baby a breast, a snack, a nap, or a diaper change. Drink even when you're awakened for a feeding in the middle of the night. That way you won't wake up in the morning feeling dehydrated, which can make you even more tired and hungry than usual.

You can have an occasional glass of flavored seltzer or fruit juice (mixed with an equal amount of water so it's not too caloric) for variety. It's best to avoid sugary sodas while nursing, and especially diet sodas or drinks with artificial sweeteners. The safety of these chemicals is still poorly understood, and lactation is not a time to take chances.

A NOTE ABOUT CAFFEINE AND ALCOHOL

Be aware that coffee, tea, and alcohol will not replenish your fluids; they will actually deplete them. Many nursing mothers avoid caffeine and alcohol completely while nursing. Others opt for a moderate consumption of no more than two cups of tea or coffee per day, and an occasional glass of wine or beer. Since these beverages have diuretic effects, you'll need extra water to replenish your fluids.

For nursing moms, the general consensus is that one or two alcoholic drinks will not harm a breast-feeding baby, although there is still some dispute on this issue. Some studies have linked as little as one drink a day with slower motor development in nursing babies. There's also been some concern about the possibility of lead deposits from wines that are wrapped in foil, so avoid bottles with this type of packaging.

ALL ABOUT CALCIUM

A very intelligent colleague of mine expressed surprise when she didn't lose all her baby weight. Then she admitted she was eating a pint of premium ice cream every night! Her rationale was that she needed the calcium because she was breast-feeding. Funny how even the smartest women can fool themselves in the pursuit of pleasure.

It's true that calcium consumption is very important while breast-feeding. Still, there are less fattening (though, alas, less delicious) sources of calcium than decadent ice cream.

Calcium is crucial for ensuring healthy bone and teeth formation in babies who are depending on breast milk. Calcium also enables muscles and nerves to work properly and is involved in blood clotting and regulating blood pressure. The recommended consumption is 1200 mg. per day for nursing moms (400 mg. more than for other women).

If you don't consume enough calcium during lactation, your body will release calcium from your bones to provide enough in the breast milk. This amazing survival mechanism protects the baby, but can put you at risk for osteoporosis later in life. So it's essential to consume adequate calcium through food sources, and through supplementation if needed.

Some Smart Calcium-rich Food Selections

FOOD/PORTION	AMOUNT OF CALCIUM
Broccoli, ½ cup	89 mg.
Calcium-fortified cereal, 1 ounce	200 mg.

FOOD/PORTION	AMOUNT OF CALCIUM
Calcium-fortified orange juice, ¾ cup	225 mg.
Cheddar cheese, 1 ounce	204 mg.
Collard greens, 1 cup cooked	300 mg.
Cottage cheese, 4 ounces	77 mg.
Kale, 1½ cups cooked	310 mg.
Milk, 1% or 2%, 1 cup	312 mg.
Milk, nonfat (skim), 1 cup	300 mg.
Sardines with bones, 3 ounces	300 mg.
Spinach, 1 cup cooked	165 mg.
Tofu, 8 ounces	300 mg.
Yogurt, flavored, nonfat, 1 cup	315–350 mg.
Yogurt, plain, nonfat, 1 cup	400–450 mg.

NOTE: You may want to select organic brands of milk and yogurt while nursing.

If it doesn't seem feasible to get all the required calcium from food sources, consider supplementation. Regular multivitamin/mineral preparations contain some calcium, but usually not enough for lactating women (check the label). Calcium carbonate supplements are another source. A supplement of 600 mg. of calcium taken with meals should suffice, in addition to some calcium foods. Consult your doctor before taking calcium supplements if you have a history of kidney stones.

VITAMIN/MINERAL SUPPLEMENTS

In the real world, it's difficult to guarantee ideal nutrition. Even when we select foods carefully, modern agricultural techniques, soil content, and freshness factors make it hard to determine the exact nutritional quality of what we are eating. Considering all the variables, it's wise to take a high-quality multivitamin/mineral supplement for insurance.

If you're breast-feeding, you'll want to be especially careful about the quality of your supplement. Many women continue to take the vitamins that their ob/gyns prescribed during pregnancy throughout the postpartum period. These prenatal formulations can provide an excellent balance of nutrients for nursing moms.

If you choose an over-the-counter supplement, learn to be a discerning label reader. The label should contain a list of nutrients and the percentage of the recommended dietary allowances (RDA) provided, although you'll have to compare this with the RDA for breast-feeding women, below, which is more in some cases. Supplements formulated specifically for pregnant and lactating women usually meet the increased demands for certain nutrients.

Recommended Dietary Allowances (RDAs) for Nursing Women

NUTRIENT	RDA
Protein	65 g.
Vitamin A	1300 mcg. RE
Vitamin D	10 mcg.
Vitamin E	12 mg.

NUTRIENT	RDA
Vitamin K	95 mcg.
Vitamin C	70 mg.
Thiamine	1.6 mg.
Riboflavin	1.8 mg.
Niacin	20 mg.
Vitamin B6	2.1 mg.
Folate	280 mcg.
Vitamin B12	2.6 mcg.
Calcium	1200 mg.
Phosphorus	1200 mg.
Magnesium	355 mg.
Iron	15 mg.
Zinc	19 mg.
Iodine	200 mcg.
Selenium	75 mcg.

HERBAL AND PHARMACEUTICAL MEDICINES

If you need to take any over-the-counter or prescription drugs during lactation, consult your physician for advice. The general rule is to not take any medication unless you must. This means no diet pills, herbal or otherwise.

Herbs can be a wonderful health aid, but they are also power-ful medicine. They can be transferred through breast milk and the consequent effect on babies' health is not sufficiently researched. Unless you are working with an experienced herbalist and are com-mitted to herbal medicine, play it safe. You can get your body back through sensible diet and exercise, without the risk of other sub-stances in your breast milk.

EXERCISE FOR THE NURSING MOM

Research on the effects of exercise on lactation brings glowing reports. Get on your sneakers and go for it . . . it's good for you and your baby!

A study at the University of California followed breast-feeding women with babies who were 9 to 24 weeks old. Half of these women participated in aerobic activity (swimming, biking, or jogging) five days a week for forty-five minutes. The other half of the women were sedentary (or as sedentary as a new mom can be). The results: The very active mothers had higher milk volumes than the sedentary women. Their milk samples were also found to be highly nutritious.

There was another interesting finding. The exercising mothers consumed 2700 calories per day and expended about 3200. The nonexercising women ate about 2100 calories and expended about 2400. So while exercising may make you hungrier, it will also help you burn calories and convert fat into muscle. And it shouldn't have any ill effects on your milk production.

Let's also dispel the old wives' tale that exercising makes breast milk sour and turns babies off feeding. Research reports that babies do not consume less breast milk when mothers exer-cise. So the little ones must be satisfied with the taste of an active mother's milk.

One caveat: Make sure your breasts are well-supported during exercise. If you're nursing, your breasts are probably larger than usual and you'll need good support to prevent sagging. Experiment to see what works for you: a sports bra or a supportive nursing bra. Some women find it's optimal to wear both while exercising (the sports bra over the nursing bra). Look for cotton bras with wide straps for extra comfort.

Nurse your baby before you start your walk or workout. If you're taking baby for a long walk, wear a style of clothing that will allow you to nurse again along the way if necessary.

BREAST-FEEDING FOR BODY AND SOUL

Breast-feeding can be a meditative, relaxing experience and an opportunity to practice relaxation techniques such as deep breathing (see page 122) or imagery. When else will you be compelled to sit down and relax for 20 minutes or so? Use this precious downtime for deep breathing, relaxing the various parts of your body, speaking positive messages to yourself and your baby.

Here is a visualization you can do while nursing that will enhance your commitment to the Get Your Body Back Program:

Visualize the healthy foods you've been eating being synthesized into nourishing breast milk, with its miraculous perfect mixture of ingredients. Feel your very life and love flowing into your baby's lips, linking you forever, nourishing her body and soul.

Feel the strength in your body that's building up through exercise. Experience how this gives your baby a sense of security and solidity in your arms.

Affirm the commitment to nourishing your body and

your baby with positive food choices. See your actions as a direct expression of love and respect for the precious baby who is taking nourishment from you. Know that you're doing the very best you can for both of you; you should be very proud.

PART TWO

THE
GET YOUR BODY BACK
PROGRAM

CHAPTER 5

READY, SET, GO:

Getting Prepared for the Program

Hopefully, by now you're excited about the program and motivated to get started. But perhaps there is still that nagging worry: How will I find time?! It seems as if all your waking moments (and many sleepless nights) are devoted to caring for your baby. And when you do get a minute to yourself, you may be so tired that all you want to do is sleep, sleep, sleep.

That's why this program is created especially for the time-crunched mommy. You can do most of the steps while caring for your baby full-time, or juggling work and childcare. Every step of the way, the realities of motherhood are addressed.

YOU DESERVE IT

If you're like most loving mothers, you probably spend a huge percentage of your time thinking about how to keep your baby happy and healthy. In the process, you may have gotten out of the habit of thinking about yourself. Perhaps you even feel vaguely guilty about spending time, thought, and energy on your own well-being.

Try to acknowledge that you do deserve a little loving attention of your own. You've given life and love to another human being—the most important act in the world. You've devoted every ounce of love and energy to making this little person flourish. And you are the whole world to your baby. You're just as important to him as he is to you.

You are the center of the family universe and you have to feel well to make it thrive. When Mommy feels good, the family is happy and secure. So never begrudge yourself the relatively small amount of time that this program requires. This effort is for you, but it also benefits everyone else in your family. It will enable you to be a more cheerful, playful, and confident mom.

SET REALISTIC GOALS

Nothing is more encouraging than success. So it's crucial to set realistic goals for the program.

Begin by creating a "Preprogram Record." Step on a digital scale when you wake up, before eating or drinking anything. The middle of your menstrual cycle will give you the most accurate reading. Write down your weight.

Then measure your chest, waistline, hips, and thighs, and record these measurements along with your current dress and pant size. This record will be useful for measuring both your weight loss and your progress as you tone and sculpt your body through exercise.

Preprogram Record

Current weight
(upon waking)_____

Chest (across bust)_____

Waist_____

Hips (widest point)_____

Thighs (widest point)_____

Dress size_____

Pant size_____

Prepregnancy weight_____

Desired weight_____
(if different than prepregnancy weight)

Look at the difference between your current weight and prepregnancy weight. If you are looking at a difference of 10 to 20 pounds, you have a good chance of losing most of the extra weight by the end of three months. A loss of 1 to 2 pounds per week is a reasonable expectation, although metabolism and genetics make it impossible to predict precisely.

Keep in mind that if you're nursing, a few extra pounds from breast fat and milk stores is likely to stay on until your baby is weaned. Mothers whose babies are being fed primarily by breast milk should not plan to lose more than a pound a week.

In case this rate of weight loss doesn't sound fast enough, consider that when weight comes off gradually, it is more likely to stay off. Severe dieting and "fad" dieting may cause rapid weight loss, but the effect will be temporary and there can be a backlash.

Research has shown that it's imperative to diet slowly and sensibly for lasting results. One study at the University of California Los Angeles showed that when a person consumes fewer than 1000 calories a day, metabolic rate slows by up to 40 percent. Slowing metabolism is the opposite of what you want to achieve if you're interested in weight control!

Another danger is that severe dieting can trigger a response where your body learns to store *more* fat. Researchers at Cedars-Sinai Medical Center found that low-calorie dieting doubled the number of lipogenic storage enzymes, which help store fat. This means that fat cells can become bigger, stronger, and more efficient at storing fat—a highly negative outcome.

Although it's tempting to succumb to the promise of "lose 10 pounds in 10 days" and other seductive fad diets, let your common sense prevail. If it's too fast and easy, do you really think it will work? Sorry, but if anyone had discovered the secret of fast, effortless, and *permanent* weight loss, the entire educated world would be slim and trim. A methodical, moderate approach is the only realistic one.

When you start the program, a reasonable goal is your prepregnancy weight, although you might be pleasantly surprised by losing even more. If your desired weight is less than your prepregnancy weight you can repeat the steps of the program for another three months for continued weight loss. But for now, go easy on yourself and your expectations and you'll set yourself up for success.

Since you'll be exercising throughout the three months, you may be gaining some pounds in muscle as you lose pounds and inches in fat. Therefore, the weigh-in alone does not provide a complete barometer of your progress. I suggest you weigh yourself only once a month. That way you'll see more progress and avoid becoming obsessed by fluctuations.

A preprogram portrait is also be a useful way to measure your progress. Have someone take a full-body, standing photo of you in form-fitting clothes. You might want to include your baby in the picture, but don't position her strategically to cover your heavy areas. When Belinda was a baby, I found that holding her in front of my tummy in photographs provided great camouflage—but it didn't fool anyone seeing me in person.

What other goals in addition to weight loss and toning can you expect to achieve in the next three months? You'll increase your energy and strength through healthy eating and exercise. You'll elevate your mood, improve your body image, and boost your self-esteem. And you'll learn little ways to treat yourself so that it's easier to cope with the world's hardest and most rewarding job: being a terrific mom.

FIND A PROGRAM PARTNER

The program in this book is designed so that you can follow it on your own. However, if you have a friend who would like to lose weight and gain fitness with you, it will be a plus.

Perhaps you have a friend or neighbor who had a baby the same year as you did. Or there's a woman from your Lamaze class, local baby playgroup, or childcare facility who might be interested. It's ideal if you can find a program partner who has a baby near the same age as yours. You'll be able to support each other in these ways:

- Giving each other encouragement to stay on the plan.

- Going food shopping together for the meal plan ingredients.

- Taking fitness walks together with the babies.

- Having the babies play together in a playpen or on the floor while you do an exercise videotape together.

- Trading off baby-sitting so your partner can enjoy a Mommy Care activity, take an exercise class, or go out for a "grown-up" evening.

- Checking weigh-ins and progress together.

- Going shopping for workout clothes and reward clothes after you lose weight.

Although it would be ideal, your program partner doesn't have to be someone with a baby. Any friend or relative (including your husband) who wants to get fit can participate.

When you're looking for a partner, show people this book and share your enthusiasm. But don't try to convince anyone who is resistant to join you because she may hold you back. Everyone has her own comfort level about weight, diet, exercise, and change. Look for someone who's motivated and optimistic about success. And if there's no one who fits that bill, you can do perfectly well on your own.

REMOVE TEMPTATION

Being with your baby is divine, but let's face it, mothering can also be tedious. If you're marooned with your baby in a house full of tempting foods, it's going to be very hard to stay on the HELP for Moms diet. Willpower is wonderful, but in the real world the siren call of the ice cream in the refrigerator or the chocolate cookies in the pantry can be irresistible.

Your program will be a lot easier and more successful if your purge your house of too-tempting foods before you start. Here's a list of potential troublemakers:

- Ice cream

- Cake, pastries, doughnuts, cookies

- Candy

- Potato chips, tortilla chips

- Cheese

What other high-fat foods do you tend to overeat? Muffins, biscuits, sweet cereals, and puddings may be other foods that you are better off purging for the duration of the program. Also consider ridding your refrigerator of caloric beverages such as soda, alcohol, and fruit drinks (other than pure fruit juices diluted with water, which you can have in a limited amount).

Be forewarned: You may encounter resistance from family members during this purging process. If you have older children who are accustomed to having sweets and chips galore, this is a good time to try to re-educate their palates. There will be protest, but the whole family will be better off if they get accustomed to having nutritious snacks instead of junk food. If this sounds like too dramatic a change, compromise by telling your children they can have these treats when they go out, but not in the house.

Your husband or other adults living in your home might also raise a ruckus when you start to throw away their favorite sweets and snacks. Here's where you'll require all your persuasive skills. Tell your partner that this program will help you regain your energy and self-esteem, as well as your figure.

Suggest a trial period of two weeks. After that, he may find he's not missing these foods, or you may find that you're ready to resist temptation. If this is absolutely unacceptable, don't be embarrassed to ask him to hide these foods from you for the duration of the diet. Out of sight, out of mind.

If the storm of protest from children, husbands, or other people who share your kitchen is too overwhelming, you may elect to leave the suspect foods in place. You'll have to exert more willpower, but after the first few weeks it should become easier. With enough commitment, you'll still be able to get your body back and feel your best.

FAMILY SUPPORT

You might expect that your spouse, family and friends would be thrilled that you're determined to get in shape. But you might be in for a disappointment. Resistance from people who are close to you can come in many forms.

If your husband loves to eat and is accustomed to lavish meals and large portions, he may be alarmed at the word "diet." There are various strategies for handling this resistance:

- The meal plan dinners are designed for four servings, but they're small ones. If he's feeling deprived, you can measure out your serving, then let him eat as much as he wants.

- Let him eat out with a friend or relative once or twice a week if he wants to indulge a taste for high-calorie, fat-laden feasts.

- Remind him that the program lasts for only three months, and then meals can become more flexible.

- In a nice way, tell him how great he'll feel and how handsome he'll look if he gets in shape along with you (assuming he could lose a few pounds, too).

- Tell him you want to get back to the size you were when you got married.

- Tell him that eating lightly and exercising may increase your libido.

Some lucky women have partners who say, "You don't need to lose weight. You look great." My own darling husband was so blinded by love he insisted that I looked the same as when we married, even though I was clearly carrying around an extra 10 pounds of baby weight.

If you have a starry-eyed spouse, don't destroy his illusions. You don't have to insist that you're fat or point out his error by trying on your wedding dress. Tell him that you appreciate his affection and find him wildly attractive, too. But you don't feel as energetic, fit, strong, or sexy as you could. Tell him that doing this will make you feel better, without emphasizing the need for weight loss or putting yourself down.

Children might be a little upset by the change in your routine. Don't focus on losing weight or getting down to a certain number on the scale when you're explaining the program to them. You don't want to create or exacerbate any worries about their own weight that can evolve into eating disorders later on. Instead, concentrate on all the benefits of eating healthfully and exercising.

You may be surprised to encounter resistance from your close friends or relatives. Sometimes people feel guilty or threatened by someone else's self-improvement efforts. The implied message is: "You should do something about your own body," which can be unnerving. If you run into defensiveness, simply say it's a personal choice and change the subject. What you do with your body is your business.

Don't waste time trying to convert doomsayers who predict that the program won't work. They're probably being negative in self-defense because they're not motivated to get in shape. The proof is in the pudding. They'll be convinced when they see how terrific you look and feel three months from now.

CHECK WITH YOUR DOCTOR

Before starting the program, obtain approval from your ob/gyn and general physician. If possible, show your doctors the meal plans and the exercise recommendations. Ascertain that you have no conditions, complications, or physical limitations to consider before starting either the workouts or the eating recommendations.

If you have undiagnosed low thyroid function, this condition can impede your progress. Please ask your physician if thyroid testing is appropriate.

If you're nursing full-time, speak with the baby's pediatrician as well as your own doctor. Your pediatrician should glance at the diet and confirm that it will be sufficient for any special nutritional needs your baby might have. In addition, work with your pediatrician to monitor your baby's weight as you slim down. The goal (and the way nature intends) is that you lose slowly, baby gains steadily, and everyone thrives.

In addition to receiving medical approval, remember to consider your emotional health before starting the program. Review the signs of postpartum depression discussed in Chapter 2. If you have any of these symptoms or signs of another mood disorder, see a mental health professional. Addressing your emotional well-being will put you in the right frame of mind for success.

If, at any time during the program, you have any illness, distress, weakness, or allergic symptoms, check with your doctor. It's unlikely that the meal plans would cause any such problems, but it's always wise to check with a health care professional.

Also be careful of overdoing the exercise if you're not accustomed to being active. If you experience any pain, injury, breathing difficulties, dizziness, or any other distress during the workouts, stop immediately and consult a doctor.

WHEN TO START

You must be a minimum of eight weeks postpartum before you start the program, and you must have your doctors' approval. Start on a Sunday to make the meal plans easy to follow. After that, it's up to you. If you're feeling sufficiently recovered, rested, and able to think clearly two months after delivery, there is no harm in starting the program then. But it may take another month or two before you're ready to tackle anything new.

Three months after delivery is often the optimal time to start the Get Your Body Back Program. By then you'll know how many extra pounds have evaporated without effort. You'll be able to assess where you are and how far you have to go to recover your prepregnancy figure.

Hopefully, your baby will have settled down somewhat by three months and be sleeping longer periods at night. Colic and other problems of infancy should be resolved. You'll have mastered diapering, feeding, and entertaining the baby. You'll feel a little less foggy and your emotions will have settled down.

When or if you go back to work is also a factor in deciding when to start. Going back to work, whether it's at six weeks or three months postpartum, is always difficult. Learning to leave your baby with a childcare provider, managing the logistics, and getting used to your "double-shift" existence is plenty to cope with at once. So don't plan to start the program when you first go back to work. Give yourself two or three weeks to get acclimated.

Realistically, however, even though three to six months postpartum is the ideal time to get started, you might not be emotionally ready at this stage. If you're still utterly exhausted, be easy on yourself. Try to eat sensibly and exercise, but give yourself a little leeway about starting a structured program. Start when you feel at least partially adjusted to motherhood.

You may be well beyond the six-month mark before you even acknowledge the need for a diet plan. It's all too easy to keep wearing those forgiving stretch pants and casual loose dresses, especially if you're staying home. It may be baby's first birthday before you face the reality that the weight isn't melting off. That's fine. It's never too late to get started.

STICK TO YOUR STARTING DATE

It's important to set a definite date to begin the program, and once you pick your date, to take it seriously. Circle it on your calendar. Tell your friends and family that's when you're starting. Honor this commitment as you do your other responsibilities. Don't let anything except a major event interfere with your starting date, or it might recede into the endless future.

SHOPPING FOR THE PROGRAM

Before starting the program, you'll need to stock up. Bring a written list with you to the supermarket. Talk to your baby as you shop to keep him amused and let him know you're excited about your new eating plan. Instill early on that the supermarket is a fun place to go and it will make your life with baby easier for a long time to come.

In the following chapters, you'll find shopping cart lists for all the ingredients required for at least the first week of each month. In the following weeks you may only have to replenish the fresh fruits, vegetables, meat, fish, and dairy products; there may be staples, spices, etc., left over. Also keep a few healthy frozen dinners on hand for nights when you're too tired or busy to cook.

If you're not confident about the quality of your tap water. I recommend buying a good filtering system instead of lugging heavy jugs of bottled water home from the market. There are a wide range of filters available, from a simple attachment to a water pitcher to under-the-sink systems. Some of the basic water filtering systems are available right at the supermarket. If you prefer bottled water, you'll need 3½ gallons a week (nonnursing) to 4½ gallons a week (nursing).

Don't forget your multivitamin/mineral supplement. The easiest way to ensure you're getting a good formula is to continue with your pregnancy vitamins. Otherwise, look for supplements that supply 100 percent or more of the U.S. RDAs. Select a special formulation if you're breast-feeding, since nursing moms require more of certain vitamins and minerals.

WORKABLE WORKOUT GEAR

The number-one aerobic exercise that moms and babies can share is fitness walking. Here's all it requires:

- Good walking shoes or sneakers
- Flexible clothes suitable for the climate, and a well-fitting sports bra
- Cozy cover-ups for your baby
- Basic diaper-bag gear
- A stroller or carriage that's suitable for the terrain

A word about fitness walking with a front-body carrier or baby backpack: Don't. These carriers can be useful when you need your hands free, and therefore fine for short excursions. But they can cause back or neck strain if you're walking briskly for a longer period of time. I know of several new moms who gamely set out with their babies strapped to their bosom, and ended up with back pain. Unless you have terrific upper-body strength and you're an experienced backpacker/hiker, you're better off pushing than carrying.

STROLLERS AND CARRIAGES FOR FITNESS WALKING

You've probably already been faced with a dizzying array of stroller choices. Let's compare them from a fitness-walking standpoint.

TRADITIONAL CARRIAGE OR PRAM. Everyone loves to see a precious baby swaddled in bunting, nestled in an grand old-fashioned pram. However, these heavyweights are not practical for fitness walking. The weight alone (about 28 pounds) is a problem, and they are cumbersome and difficult to maneuver. If you have such a carriage, enjoy a promenade on a sunny day, but pick up a different model for long walks.

JOGGING STROLLERS. Three-wheeled jogging strollers are great for fast-moving moms. But you have to be sure a jogging stroller is also comfortable for your baby. Jogging strollers aren't practical for newborns because the seats don't fully recline. And some older babies don't like the low, somewhat "slouchy" seating they provide. Unless you're planning to run, rather than walk, or to walk on bumpy terrain, a jogger stroller is probably not necessary.

CONVERTIBLE STROLLERS. These multi-use strollers come in many sizes, models, and prices. Many have reclining and upright positions, so they can be used for infants and for older babies, who want to sit up and see the world. Some have toy bars, juice and snack trays, and other doodads. You definitely want to select a model that reclines—no baby should be discouraged from sleeping while you're getting exercise! Also look for a sunshade and a basket to store your bottles, diapers, and diversions. Choose a style that's sturdy and comfy for baby, but fairly lightweight.

UMBRELLA STROLLERS. These strollers get their name from the umbrella-like way they can be folded up and carried. They are lighter and more maneuverable than most convertible strollers, and quite versatile. Some of the better models fully recline, a desirable feature.

CAR SEAT STROLLERS. These inventions consist of a car seat that can be removed from the vehicle, then snapped into place on top of a wheeled contraption to create a stroller. They are supposed to be convenient, but many mothers find them hard to manipulate. You'll probably want to save this style for car excursions, where it offers the advantage of allowing you to transfer a sleeping baby without unstrapping him. For everyday fitness walks, a simple, inexpensive stroller is easier to handle.

DOUBLE STROLLERS. If you have twins or two young children, you'll need a double stroller for a fitness walk of any sustained length. No matter how energetic, a toddler or preschooler can't be trusted to walk briskly for half an hour or more. What you'll discover is that most young children have a one-way trajectory. They will walk quite a distance one way, then demand to be carried on the return journey.

If you're shopping for a double stroller, you have two options: side-by-side or tandem. In the tandem strollers, one child sits behind the other, and in some models the seat flips to a face-to-face position. Side-by-side strollers have horizontal seating, and their width makes them hard to maneuver on narrow sidewalks. Tandem strollers are more practical for fitness walking, but even these can be very heavy. You may have to moderate your workout accordingly until you build up muscle and endurance.

SHOPPING FOR THE FITNESS-FRIENDLY STROLLER

Look for these features:

- A reclining seat and sun shade so that baby is comfortable and protected

- Stability and large enough wheels for good maneuverability

- Reliable restraining belts and locking mechanism for baby's safety

- Fairly light weight (10–12 pounds)

- A handlebar that is the right height for you

You do enough hunching and bending when you're caring for your baby—don't add stress to your fitness walk. The wrong height handle can strain your neck, upper back, and shoulders. Be sure to do a "test drive" before purchasing the stroller to see if it is suitable.

The correct height allows your arms to be bent at approximately a 120-degree angle, your shoulders to remain relaxed and open, and your upper body straight. If your arms are bent at a 90-degree angle, the handlebar is too high. If your arms are almost straight and your shoulders are hunched over the stroller, the handlebar is too low. For the best results, check your form in a mirror in the store using the display model.

SHOES AND CLOTHING FOR FITNESS WALKING

Okay, you have your stroller, you have your baby; the essential item is a pair of supportive, well-cushioned shoes. These can be fitness shoes or sneakers that are designed for "cross training" or walking. The shoes should be big enough to accommodate a pair of cushy sports socks. Before warned that you may need a larger size than you did before getting pregnant.

Your feet aren't the only part of your body that needs extra support now that you're a mom. Your breasts need consideration, especially if you're nursing. Take the bounce test while walking briskly in your usual bra. If your breasts jiggle at all, you need more support.

Sports bras are usually a safe bet. However, if you're nursing, a sports bra alone may not be supportive enough. Many women wear a sports bra over a nursing bra. Before you laugh, consider the advantage: If you need to feed your baby while out and about you can find a discreet spot, lift up the sports bra, unhook the nursing bra, and voilá.

When it comes to clothing, you have free range. Just be sure that your clothes are comfortable, flexible, and cozy, but not stuffy. Don't forget gloves for chilly days. On sunny days, you'll need sunglasses and sunscreen.

DRESSING BABY

Dress your baby warmly enough, but don't overbundle or he might get fussy. Have him wear a sunhat on hot days and a hat that covers his ears on cold days. If he's over six months old, you can use a baby sunscreen on bright days. Bring a stroller blanket along for snuggling. Add a spare outfit if your baby's prone to diaper leaks or massive spit-ups.

OTHER ITEMS FOR THE WALK

- Two diapers and a small plastic bag of wipes, plus a regular-size plastic bag for disposal or dirty diapers

- A blanket or changing pad

- One or two bottles of milk and/or juice (or your breasts)

- Two pacifiers, if your baby uses them (one may fall on the ground)

- A cuddly toy to encourage sleeping

- A bottle of water for you

Either pack these items in the diaper bag, or put them in the basket at the bottom of the stroller—and you're ready to roll.

FALLING OFF THE WAGON

The Get Your Body Back Program will give you optimal results if you follow it to the letter. But chances are, you won't. You're human. You're busy. Temptations lurk all around you. You're bound to succumb once or twice to a cheesy baked ziti, a gift of French chocolates, or a pile of chips and dips at a party. No one expects you to be perfect, especially when you're working so hard at being the perfect mom.

If you fall off the wagon and diverge from the meal plans, it's not a big problem—as long as you don't use it as an excuse to give up. Don't berate yourself. Don't shrug your shoulders and say that it's hopeless. Just go right back to the menus, and you'll hardly see a blip in the screen (or scale).

The same applies to exercise. There may be times when your baby is teething and keeps you up all night. Or the poor little sweetie has a fever and you're marooned. Or you're trying to meet a work deadline and you can't take time out for exercise despite your desire. Again, don't wallow in guilt and give up in despair. Simply return to your exercise routine as soon as you possibly can.

Fitness is not an all-or-nothing-at-all proposition. Doing most or even some of the steps of this program is better than doing nothing. Sticking with it 90 percent of the time is better than giving up.

READY, SET, GO: ACTION STEPS

1. Fill out your Preprogram Record (see page 76). Also have a full-body picture of yourself taken in form-fitting clothes for later comparison.

2. Purge your kitchen of diet-sabotaging foods such as ice cream, cake, candy, cookies, pastries, doughnuts, and chips.

3. Find a program partner, if you want one.

4. Explain to your family and close friends what you'll be doing and why it's important to you, to gather their support.

5. Check with your doctor and your baby's pediatrician (if you're nursing) to ascertain that the eating and exercise recommendations are safe and suitable for you.

6. Get yourself a fitness-friendly stroller, good sports shoes or sneakers, and comfortable walking clothes.

7. Set a date to get started. Unless something drastic happens, stick with that date.

CHAPTER 6

MONTH 1:

Meal Plans, Workouts, and Mommy Care

Congratulations on getting started. This month you will notice gratifying results as you consume a slimming diet, build your stamina through regular exercise, and pay attention to your personal needs.

As explained earlier, seven days of meal plans are provided for each month. After the first week, repeat these meal plans for the remaining three weeks of the month. This system is designed to make the program simpler for you to follow. The recipes will become familiar and the routine of preparing light, easy meals will require less effort.

If you want more variety or dislike any of the choices on the meal plans, you can substitute foods from other days occasionally. For example, if you don't care for fish, substitute a meat dinner. If you can't stand cottage cheese, replace it with a yogurt. If you want cold cereal with milk for breakfast instead of oatmeal, no problem. As long as you select choices from other meal plans within the program, you'll be staying within the parameters of low-fat foods with high nutritional value.

When you're really harried and don't have the time or energy to cook even the simplest dinner, you can substitute a low-fat prepared frozen dinner (less than 350 calories). But try not to do this more than once a week, since frozen foods are not as nutritious as fresh.

Many of the meal plans include a dessert to satisfy your sweet tooth. But if you don't desire sweets, or you're feeling especially virtuous, you can always substitute fresh fruit for the suggested dessert.

Have your first meal less than a half hour after you wake up and space your subsequent meals out every two to three hours. Try to sit down, relax, and enjoy your food (if the baby allows it). Eat your dinner by 6:30 P.M., with the option of saving your dessert for a little later.

Don't forget to add sufficient breast-feeding bonus foods if you're nursing. And take a high-quality multivitamin/mineral supplement everyday.

Drink eight to ten glasses of water per day. If there is no beverage indicated on the meal plan, have a glass of water with that meal.

SHOPPING CART LIST: MONTH 1

This list contains all the foods you need to purchase for at least one week's worth of meal plans. At the beginning of the following weeks, you'll need to replenish supplies of produce, dairy products, meat, and fish. But you will have extra stores of condiments, grains, and snacks. The easiest way to manage shopping is a two step process:

1. Before starting the program, stock your kitchen with everything on the list.

2. The 2nd, 3rd, and 4th weeks of the first month, use this master list to make a fresh list of everything you need to replenish.

Keep in mind that there are many variable factors—especially the other people in your house. You might find that a box of cookies is gone although you had only two. You might discover that your yogurt is used up before you get to it on the meal plan. Try to take these factors into consideration when you're shopping. At any rate, you can also go back to the store to refresh your supplies. Meanwhile, the shopping cart lists will get you off to a good start.

PRODUCE
Apple, 1
Asparagus spears, fresh (20 spears) or 1 8-ounce package frozen
Bananas, 2
Blueberries, fresh or frozen, 1 pint
Broccoli florets, fresh (1 head) or frozen (1 10-ounce package)
Cantaloupe, 1
Carrots, fresh baby, 1-pound bag
Celery, 1 bunch
Garlic, 1 bulb
Grapes, red or green, small bunch
Grapefruit, 2
Lemon, 2
Lemon juice, 1 small bottle
Mushrooms, fresh button, 1 10-ounce package
Onions, white, 4 small
Oranges, 3
Pears, 3 fresh or pear halves, 1 15-ounce can
Peppermint, fresh, small bunch
Plum, 1
Potatoes, white russet, 1 5-pound bag
Salad, prewashed blend of your choice, 2 bags

Snap beans, fresh (4 cups) or frozen, 1 package
Spinach, fresh or frozen, 1 package
Sweet potatoes, 2 medium
Tomatoes, 5 large fresh

DAIRY
Butter, light, 1 8-ounce container
Buttermilk, light, 32 ounces
Cheese, cheddar low-fat, 8 ounces
Cheese, cheddar low-fat and shredded, 8-ounce bag
Cheese, grated Parmesan, 8 ounces
Cheese, mozzerella low-fat and shredded, 8-ounce bag
Cottage cheese, low-fat, 1 pound
Cream cheese, light, 8 ounces
Eggs, 1 dozen
Egg product, Egg Beaters, 16 ounces
Milk, nonfat (organic recommended if you're nursing), 1 gallon
Pudding, chocolate nonfat, 6 4-ounce cups
Yogurt, low-fat fruit flavor, 1 8-ounce container
Yogurt, low-fat frozen, peach or flavor of choice, 1 pint

MEAT/FISH

Chicken breasts, boneless, 2 pounds

Chicken breast, chunky, 2 10-ounce cans

Beef flank, 1 pound

Fish fillets of choice, 4 4-ounce fillets of orange roughy, flounder, or cod

Ham lunch meat, nonfat 40% ham/water, 8-ounce package

Pork, 4 4-ounce loin chops

Sole fillet, 1 pound

Tuna, 1 12-ounce can in water

Turkey breast, sliced, ¼ pound

Turkey, lean ground, 1 pound

GRAINS

Bagel, 1 small

Bread, Pepperidge Farm garlic bread (frozen)

Bread, pita, whole wheat, small, 1 package

Bread, multigrain, 1 loaf

Bread, oat bran reduced-calorie, 1 loaf

Bread, French, 1 loaf

Bread, whole wheat hamburger buns, 1 package of 4

Breadcrumbs, Italian

Cereal, hot, multigrain, 1 box of instant packets

Cereal, Kellogg's All Bran

Cereal, Kellogg's Special K

Cereal bars, Nutrigrain Smart Start, strawberry

Cornmeal, white, 1 2-pound bag

Crackers, Snack Well's Classic Golden Crackers, reduced fat, 1 box

English muffins, 1 package

Flour, white wheat all purpose, 2 pounds

Oatmeal, H-O whole grain instant, 1 pound

Pancake mix, light, 1 box

Rice, brown medium grain instant, 1 box

Rice, white long grain, 1 pound

Spaghetti, 1 1-lb. package

SPICES, CONDIMENTS, SAUCES, OIL

Basil, ground

Bean dip, Bearitos nonfat vegetarian, 1 small jar

Canola oil spray

Celery salt

Cinnamon, ground

Dill weed, dried

Garlic powder

Ginger, ground

Horseradish

Hot pepper sauce

Lemon pepper seasoning

Ketchup

Mayonnaise, light, 1 16-ounce jar

Mustard

Mustard powder

Nutmeg, ground
Onion powder
Pepper, ground black
Pancake syrup, light
Paprika
Parsley
Pickle relish, sweet
Preserves, blueberry
Salad dressing, diet French
Salad dressing, low-fat
  Thousand Island
Salsa, mild, 1 jar
Salt
Soy sauce, low sodium, or
  teriyaki sauce, light
Spaghetti sauce, garden style,
  1 26-ounce jar
Tarragon, fresh or dried
Thyme, ground
Vinegar, red wine
Vegetable oil spread, 40% oil,
  1 8-ounce container (or
  light butter if you prefer)
Worcestershire sauce

MISC.
Apple juice, ½ gallon
Brownies, Weight Watcher's
  frozen, 1 package
Cookies, Health Valley granola
Cookies, Snack Well's
  chocolate chip
Chocolate covered mints,
  1 small box

Cornstarch
Orange juice, with calcium
  added, ½ gallon
Pine nuts, 1 small package
Popcorn, Gourmet microwave
  light butter-flavored
Raisins, bag of miniature
  boxes
Sherry, dry
Soup, Healthy Choice Country
  Garden Vegetable,
  1 15-ounce can
Soup, Healthy Choice
  Minestrone, 1 15-ounce can
Soup, Swanson 99% fat free
  chicken broth, 1 32-ounce
  can or carton
Vegetable juice, V-8,
  1 46-ounce container
Whipped topping, light,
  1 8-ounce container

OPTIONAL/AS NEEDED
Additional breast-feeding
  bonus foods
Frozen dinners, low-fat and
  low-calorie
Fresh fruit for dessert
Orange liqueur for baked pear
  dessert, 1 small bottle
Seltzer water, flavored
Water, 3½– 4½ gallons (if you
  don't have a filtering
  system)

MEAL PLANS

Month 1: Sunday

DAILY TOTALS, ALL FOODS

CALORIES	PROTEIN (G)	CARBS (G)	FAT (G)	SAT. FAT (G)	CHOL. (MG)	SODIUM (MG)	FIBER (G)
1604.51	108.86	245.56	28.35	4.01	108.45	2805.25	18.03

BREAKFAST
Banana, ½ medium
Special K cereal, 1 cup
Nonfat milk, 1 cup

MORNING MINI-MEAL
Snack Well's Classic Golden Crackers, reduced fat, 10
Cheddar cheese, low-fat, 1 ounce, sliced to put on crackers

LUNCH
Turkey Sandwich*
Orange
Tossed salad, 1½ cups
Low-fat Thousand Island dressing, 1 tablespoon
Nonfat milk, 1 cup

AFTERNOON MINI-MEAL
Cantaloupe, ¼
Nonfat cottage cheese, ½ cup

DINNER
Savory Tarragon Chicken*, 1 serving
Comforting Mashed Potatoes*, 1 serving

Broccoli spears, 4 ounces, frozen and cooked as per directions, or
fresh and steamed
Light butter or 40% vegetable oil spread
Peach frozen yogurt, low-fat, ½ cup
Chocolate chip cookie, SnackWell's, 1

*Substitute fresh fruit for dessert if desired. Add breast-feeding bonus foods (pages 60–62)
as needed—see Chapter 4.*

*See Chapter 9 for recipes.

Month 1: Monday

DAILY TOTALS, ALL FOODS

CALORIES	PROTEIN (G)	CARBS (G)	FAT (G)	SAT. FAT (G)	CHOL. (MG)	SODIUM (MG)	FIBER (G)
1518.08	101.95	235.70	22.96	4.12	47.60	3078.94	17.32

BREAKFAST
Multigrain hot cereal, instant, 1 packet
Raisins, 1 miniature box
Nonfat milk, 1 cup

MORNING MINI-MEAL
Grapefruit, ½
SnackWell's Classic Golden Crackers, reduced fat, 8

LUNCH
Chicken Salad Pita Sandwich*
Garden Vegetable Soup, Healthy Choice, 1 cup
Grapes, ½ cup, red or green
Nonfat milk, 1 cup

AFTERNOON MINI-MEAL
Strawberries, fresh or frozen and thawed, 1 cup

DINNER
Tangy Baked Dover Sole*, 1 serving
Italian Grilled Tomatoes*, 1 serving
Chinese Rice*, 1 serving
Light butter or 40% vegetable oil spread
Baby carrots, 1 cup
Chocolate chip cookie, SnackWell's, 1

Substitute fresh fruit for dessert if desired. Add breast-feeding bonus foods (pages 60–62) as needed—see Chapter 4.

*See Chapter 9 for recipes.

Month 1: Tuesday

DAILY TOTALS, ALL FOODS

CALORIES	PROTEIN (G)	CARBS (G)	FAT (G)	SAT. FAT (G)	CHOL. (MG)	SODIUM (MG)	FIBER (G)
1503.69	91.81	257.90	25.32	6.64	76.22	2587.95	37.62

BREAKFAST
All-Bran cereal, Kellogg's, ¾ cup
Raisins, 1 miniature box
Nonfat milk, 1 cup

MORNING MINI-MEAL
Deviled Eggs*, 2 servings (save leftovers for Wednesday)
Apple

LUNCH
Turkey Sandwich*
Orange
Nonfat milk, 1 cup

AFTERNOON MINI-MEAL
Baby carrots, 1 cup
Bean dip, Bearitos nonfat vegetarian, 2.5 ounces
Vegetable juice, V-8 low-salt, 1 cup

DINNER
Seasoned Stuffed Potatoes*, 1 serving
Marinated Flank Steak*, 1 serving
Snap beans, ½ cup
Tossed salad, 1½ cups
Salad dressing, nonfat creamy, 1 tablespoon
French or Vienna bread, 1 slice
Light butter or 40% vegetable oil spread, 1 tablespoon
Baked Pears au Chocolate*, 1 serving

Substitute fresh fruit for dessert if desired. Add breast-feeding bonus foods (pages 60–62) as needed—see Chapter 4.

*See Chapter 9 for recipes.

Month 1: Wednesday

CALORIES	PROTEIN (G)	CARBS (G)	FAT (G)	SAT. FAT (G)	CHOL. (MG)	SODIUM (MG)	FIBER (G)
1508.81	91.85	241.03	26.13	3.94	42.62	1719.43	21.68

BREAKFAST
Blueberry Egg White Pancakes*, 1 serving
Nonfat milk, 1 cup

MORNING MINI-MEAL
Pear
Deviled Eggs*, 2 servings (left over from Tuesday)

LUNCH
Low-fat cottage cheese, ½ cup
Strawberries, fresh or frozen and thawed, 1 cup
Oat bran bread, reduced calorie, 1 slice toasted
Light butter or 40% vegetable oil spread, 1 tablespoon

AFTERNOON MINI-MEAL
2 stalks raw celery, dipped into low-fat Thousand Island dressing, 1
   tablespoon
SnackWell's Classic Golden Crackers, reduced fat, 5

DINNER
Breaded Fish Fillet*, 1 serving
Brown rice, medium-grain instant, ½ cup cooked
Baby carrots, ½ cup
Tossed salad, 1½ cups

Salad dressing, diet French, 2 ounces

Brownie, Weight Watchers, frozen and thawed

Substitute fresh fruit for dessert if desired. Add breast-feeding bonus foods (pages 60–62) as needed—see Chapter 4.

*See Chapter 9 for recipes.

Month 1: Thursday

DAILY TOTALS, ALL FOODS

CALORIES	PROTEIN (G)	CARBS (G)	FAT (G)	SAT. FAT (G)	CHOL. (MG)	SODIUM (MG)	FIBER (G)
1501.83	120.26	222.46	20.63	5.61	145.39	3218.45	18.25

BREAKFAST
Salsa Breakfast Scramble*, 1 serving

Orange juice, 1 cup

MORNING MINI-MEAL
Oat bran bread, 1 slice toasted

Light cream cheese, 1 tablespoon

Plum

LUNCH
Lean Turkey Burgers*, 1 serving

Nonfat milk, 1 cup

AFTERNOON MINI-MEAL
Fruit Smoothie*, 1 serving

Popcorn, Gourmet microwave light butter-flavored, 3 cups

DINNER

Stuffed Chicken Breasts*, 1 serving

Asparagus spears, canned or fresh steamed, ½ cup

Tossed salad, 1½ cups

Salad dressing, nonfat creamy, ½ tablespoon

Nonfat milk, 1 cup

Granola cookies, Health Valley, 3

Substitute fresh fruit for dessert if desired. Add breast-feeding bonus foods (pages 60–62) as needed—see Chapter 4.

*See Chapter 9 for recipes.

Month 1: Friday

DAILY TOTALS, ALL FOODS

CALORIES	PROTEIN (G)	CARBS (G)	FAT (G)	SAT. FAT (G)	CHOL. (MG)	SODIUM (MG)	FIBER (G)
1519.84	94.76	246.26	17.72	5.13	111.28	3272.77	7.63

BREAKFAST

Apple-Cinnamon Grapefruit*, 1 serving

Plain bagel, small, toasted

Light cream cheese, 2 tablespoons

MORNING MINI-MEAL

Yogurt, low-fat, any fruit flavor, 8 ounces

LUNCH

Low-fat cottage cheese, 4 ounces

Cantaloupe, ¼

Nonfat milk, 1 cup

AFTERNOON MINI-MEAL

Grapes, 10

SnackWell's Classic Golden Crackers, reduced fat, 8

DINNER

Grilled Glazed Pork Chops*, 1 serving

Sweet Potato Puffs*, 1 serving

Tossed salad, 1½ cups

Diet French salad dressing, 1 tablespoon

Nonfat milk, 1 cup

Chocolate pudding, nonfat, 1 serving

Substitute fresh fruit for dessert if desired. Add breast-feeding bonus foods (pages 60–62) as needed—see Chapter 4.

*See Chapter 9 for recipes.

Month 1: Saturday

DAILY TOTALS, ALL FOODS

CALORIES	PROTEIN (G)	CARBS (G)	FAT (G)	SAT. FAT (G)	CHOL. (MG)	SODIUM (MG)	FIBER (G)
1514.17	83.50	226.45	33.84	8.94	283.00	2795.09	13.27

BREAKFAST

Scrambled egg, cooked with canola oil spray, 1

Oat bran bread, 1 slice

Light butter or 40% vegetable oil spread, ½ tablespoon

Orange

MORNING MINI-MEAL
Low-fat cottage cheese, ½ cup
Cantaloupe, ¼

LUNCH
Tuna Salad Pita Sandwich*
Healthy Choice Minestrone Soup, 1 serving
Nonfat milk, 1 cup

AFTERNOON MINI-MEAL
Nutrigrain Smart Start strawberry cereal bar

DINNER
Spaghetti, 1 cup cooked (2 ounces dry)
Spaghetti sauce, garden style, ½ cup
Parmesan cheese, grated, 1 ounce
Garlic bread, frozen Pepperidge Farm, 1 slice cooked
Nonfat milk, 1 cup
Frozen yogurt, low-fat flavor of choice, 1 cup

Substitute fresh fruit for dessert if desired. Add breast-feeding bonus foods (pages 60–62) as needed—see Chapter 4.

*See Chapter 9 for recipes.

MAKING THE MEAL PLANS WORK FOR YOU

If you work full-time outside the home, you'll need a supply of plastic containers and a small insulated food carrier so you can bring your lunches and snacks to work. If you want to be campy, you can pick out a lunchbox that makes you smile. I'm fond of my pink "I Dream of Jeannie" lunchbox, shaped like a sixties TV set.

Pack your lunch and snacks the night before so that you're not even more pressured than usual in the morning rush. If you need a break from bringing lunch, select foods from a salad bar style restaurant or deli that fit the parameters of the diet plan. But you'll have to be careful about portion control and hidden fat. Most days, it's better to prepare lunch from the meal plan and bring it to work, so you know exactly what you're getting.

DEVELOPING THE WATER HABIT

Remember to keep yourself well hydrated with plenty of water throughout the day and evening. For the first month of the program (until drinking a lot of water becomes a habit), it's good to keep track of your consumption. Put a note near the water source every day and make a mark each time you fill and finish a serving of water. To help remind yourself:

- Drink a glass every time you finish nursing or bottle-feeding your baby.

- Drink a glass whenever you put the baby down for a nap or bedtime.

- Drink a glass a half hour before each of your five mini-meals.

- Drink a glass after you exercise.

- Leave bottles of water in the nursery, the living room, and the car.

- Drink water whenever you think about eating.

MOTHER'S HELPER HINT: After 6:30 P.M., keep a bottle of water in the living room, so you don't have to venture into the kitchen, where you'll be tempted to snack.

DEVELOPING THE EATING EARLY ROUTINE

A challenging task in the first month is to establish the habit of eating your dinner by 6:30 P.M. If you are nursing, add one snack at 8 P.M. Otherwise, try to avoid nighttime eating.

There are many reasons why we succumb to nighttime eating. After a day at work, we're finally home with the food. Or the baby is in bed and we can finally sit down to a peaceful meal. Or we're accustomed to munching snacks while watching TV. Or our willpower has simply evaporated by this time because we're exhausted. But with a little advance planning you can overcome these pitfalls.

Make an effort to sit down for a relaxing breakfast or lunch. If you work outside the home, perhaps breakfast or lunch can be a social, sit-down meal. If you're at home, have your meal while the baby is napping, or let her watch a little television so you can eat in peace. A brief oasis of eating during the day will make you less desperate when night falls.

Stay out of the kitchen as much as possible after you've finished your early dinner. Play with the baby and talk on the phone in another room. Brush your teeth so that lingering flavors don't tempt you to eat more.

WORKABLE WORKOUTS FOR MONTH 1

You're going to start slow and easy, and work your way up to more aerobic intensity and variety throughout the three months. You'll do enough exercise to burn fat, rev up your metabolism, energize your cells, and brighten your mood. But unless you're so inclined, you're not expected to become a superaerobicized workout queen—just a nice, fit, and toned mom who's proud to have her body back.

You're probably already aware of the benefits of exercise and its importance in a weight-loss and fitness program. But even when you know what's good for you, it's hard to do it, especially when you're facing the twin obstacles of being tired and busy. That's why this program emphasizes workouts you can fit into your life as a mom, whether you're working or staying home, whether you have a baby-sitter or not.

FITNESS WALKING: BABY STEPS

There's a difference between everyday locomotion and walking for fitness. Although you'll be pushing the stroller, you can't merely stroll and expect major gains. There are four components to consider when you want to maximize the fitness value of walking:

- Posture

- Frequency

- Pace

- Duration

PERFECT YOUR POSTURE. You'll have to gaze down occasionally to coo at your baby and pick up a pacifier or adjust a cute hat that falls into her eyes. But don't make the mistake of looking down at your baby throughout the walk. Keep your neck long, head up, and shoulders back. Even though your hands are on the stroller bar, if it's the right height you should be able to avoid hunching.

If you're nursing, your larger-than-usual breasts might tend to pull your body forward into a slouch. The fitness walk is a good time to start correcting this tendency. Keep your shoulders relaxed and down, without letting them round. Lift your bountiful bosom proudly. It will help to prevent back and neck pain, as well as reduce the risk of sagging breasts.

Use your walk as an opportunity for tummy toning by keeping your stomach tucked in. Don't hold your breathe or tuck under too much, but keep your abdomen as firm and lifted as you can. This is a way to start regaining your abdominal tone over the next three months.

Keep your hips in line with your shoulders and facing forward. Keep your feet under your knees, closer together than the wheels of the stroller. Your toes should be pointed forward as you walk.

Be aware of the way you're holding the stroller bar. Although you want a firm grip on your precious cargo, you don't have to hold too tightly to keep control. Don't bend your wrists as you hold the stroller bar; this can lead to problems such as carpal tunnel syndrome. Instead, keep your wrists straight and your hands fairly relaxed on the handle. As long as baby's well strapped in, she's not going anywhere without you.

DEVELOP YOUR FREQUENCY, PACE, AND DURATION. Next month we'll learn an easy method for measuring your heart rate, so you can increase the aerobic challenge of your fitness walks. But for Month 1, the goal is even simpler:

Walk as often as you can, as far as you can, as fast as you can without feeling strain or pain.

The minimum requirement for fitness is to walk three times a week for 30 minutes each session. If that's absolutely impossible, walk for two 15-minutes sessions per day. Walking more than three times a week is even better. If your baby falls asleep in the stroller or is contentedly watching the scenery pass by, count your blessings and walk for more than a half hour on some days.

Always start by walking slowly or moderately for the first 5 or 10 minutes to warm up your muscles. Then increase your pace to enhance the aerobic benefits.

Walk fast enough that it feels challenging, but not so fast that you get breathless. Try the talk/sing test: You should be able to speak comfortably, but need to take extra breaths if you sing. Your heart should be beating faster than when you are sitting down or strolling slowly. But if you experience any dizziness, breathlessness, or other ill effects, slow down. And if you have any chest pain or difficulty breathing, stop and see your doctor.

Adding some hills to your walk dramatically increases the aerobic effect and helps strengthen and tone. If there's only one hill on your route, go up and down it several times during your fitness walk. Pushing the stroller uphill will help condition your upper body, hamstrings, and heart.

YOUR WALKING ROUTINE. Where and when should you walk? The answer is, wherever and whenever it's convenient for you and your baby. Most people simply set out from their homes and follow the sidewalk. For a change of perspective, drive to a scenic park.

If your baby is reasonably content in the stroller, go when he's awake, after a nap, a meal, and a diaper change. The walk is a wonderful way to pass time pleasantly together. He'll enjoy seeing the world and the world will enjoy seeing him. The only down side is that you might have to stop to let admirers look at the little cutie.

Any time during daylight hours should be fine. If you go in the morning, you'll have a better chance of getting out for a second walk in the afternoon. But keep in mind: It's best if you've had some food and water within two hours before the walk so you aren't distracted by hunger or thirst.

If you're working full-time and you don't get home until after dusk, you have two choices. If you're heroic, you can get up extra early and walk with your baby or on your own before breakfast. But personally, I don't know many mothers who would willingly give up any chance to cling to their pillows in the early morning. A more realistic plan is to walk briskly for the first half hour of your lunch hour; then eat a light meal. Leave an extra pair of walking shoes or sneakers in your office and you're set. In addition to the physical benefits, walking at lunchtime will give you a mental boost and minimize the dreaded afternoon slump.

HOW TO KEEP YOUR CHILD HAPPY DURING FITNESS WALKS

If your baby is under one year:

- Nurse or bottle-feed before going on the walk, and bring extra bottles.

- Start out with a clean diaper; bring spare diapers, wipes, and a plastic bag for disposal.

- Bring two pacifiers if you use them (in case the first one drops on the ground).

- Bring snacks once your baby is feeding herself.

- Make sure your baby is never cold, but not overdressed.

- Keep the direct sun out of the baby's eyes with a stroller sunshade and a hat when needed.

- Clamp little toys or rattles on the front bar.

- Let your baby hear your soothing voice throughout the walk.

- Play lullabies or favorite songs on a portable cassette or CD player.

If your child is one to three years:

- Be sure your baby or toddler is cozily attired but not too stuffy or hot; keep the direct sun off his face.

- Bring ample bottles of milk or formula, and later on "sippy" cups of juice or milk.

- Bring various snacks (but don't eat them yourself).

- Bring little toys and books for your child to look at and hold.

- Chat to your toddler, pointing out interesting sights along the way.

- Ask your toddler lots of questions along the way.

- Give him little tasks, such as spotting every bird he can see.

- Walk to a destination that engages your toddler, such as the playground, a duck pond, or the library (but not a fattening destination like the ice cream shop!).

When your child's over one and a half:

- Let her get out occasionally to walk alongside you, holding hands.

- Let her push the stroller for a while. Toddlers usually find this to be quite thrilling.

NOTE: As your child grows up, he might protest against sitting in the stroller. But don't be lulled into thinking that he can last through a long walk. Take the stroller along even if he thinks he's too old for it. Let him walk until he's tired; then he'll be happy to climb in the stroller and you can pick up the pace.

COOL-DOWN STRETCHES

When you're finished with your fitness walk, do the following stretches to cool down, avoid stiffness, and maintain flexibility. You can keep your baby in the stroller while you do these if he's not too restless. Or transfer him to a crib, playpen, or other comfy location at home where he can watch you.

STANDING LEG LUNGE

Stand up tall. Bring your left leg back straight and gently press your heel toward the ground as you bend your right (front) leg. Don't bounce or stretch beyond comfort. The stretch comes from pressing the back foot toward the ground gently. If you need to you can hold onto the stroller handle for balance. Hold the stretch for 30 seconds. Then bring your left (back) leg forward into a standing position. Reverse, bringing the right leg back and bending the left knee. Stretch for 30 seconds. Repeat the exercise on each side.

STANDING STRETCH

Stand with your feet hip-width apart. Lift both arms overhead. Stretch your right arm up and the right side of the body long; then the left side. Repeat 4 times. Lower your arms.

NECK AND SHOULDER STRETCH

Slowly turn your head from right to left 4 times. Drop your chin to your chest, then look up to the sky or ceiling (stretching your neck long but not letting it drop back) 4 times. Shrug your shoulders up and down 4 times. Circle your shoulders toward the back 4 times, then reverse direction and circle toward the front 4 times.

ROLLDOWN

From a standing position, drop your head, then begin to bend forward slowly, rolling your spine down. Bend your knees as you roll down if you need to, and be careful not to "lock" them as you perform this exercise. Touch the floor or wherever you can comfortably reach. Relax your back and let it lengthen. Then slowly roll up from the bottom of your spine to standing straight again, head coming up last.

QUADRICEP STRETCH

Stand tall. You can hold onto the stroller for support. Bending your right leg at the knee, lift your foot behind you, grasp hold of it, and press your heel toward your buttocks. The thigh of your bent leg should be parallel to that of your standing leg. You should feel a comfortable, not painful, stretch in your thigh and no tension in your knee. Hold for 10 seconds Slowly release your leg down until you are standing on both feet again. Then, do the same with your left leg. Repeat on both sides.

UPPER BACK STRETCH

Stand tall. Stretch your arms behind your body and clasp your hands, palms facing in. Try to straighten your arms while gently pressing your chest forward. Hold and breathe deeply for 30 seconds. This is a great release for your upper body, especially after you've been pushing the stroller.

Okay, you're done. And if you've gotten this far without your baby demanding your attention, consider yourself lucky!

INDOOR AEROBIC ALTERNATIVES

Be prepared to do an alternative aerobic workout on days when it's too rainy, snowy, or cold for a fitness walk. Some possibilities:

- Dance or run around your living room.

- Rent or buy aerobic workout videotapes (see suggestions in month 3, pages 171–74).

- Use a treadmill or exercise bicycle (see month 2, page 143).

- When your child is old enough, look for a gym with baby-sitting services.

- If you have baby-sitting coverage, head out to a class.

THE FREELANCE DANCE. If your baby is too restless to allow you to complete an exercise-machine workout or video, other types of indoor aerobic exercise may be more entertaining. Easiest of all is to pick out your favorite CD or audiotape—something with a driving percussive beat—get into your workout clothes (don't forget the sports bra), and dance, jump, and run around your living room for half an hour. I call this "the freelance dance" workout.

Pick up your baby up and rock him in your arms as you dance. Lift him up and down. Dip him upside down (carefully), whirl him around. Get down on the floor and crawl. Pretend you are a dog or a cat. Be a jack-in-the-box. Your baby will love it.

Anything goes. The only rule is that you have to keep moving for 30 minutes. If you have to stop to feed or change the baby, stop the clock and start it up again as soon as you're done. The freelance dance workout will raise your spirits, break up a long day at home, and make you feel like a little kid yourself.

WORKABLE WORKOUT MONTH 1 ACTION STEPS

1. Walk with your baby, 30 minutes per session, three times a week or more. Walk at a brisk pace and include some hills.

2. Find an alternative aerobic workout for indoor days.

3. Do the cool-down stretches after your fitness walk or aerobic exercise.

MOMMY CARE FOR MONTH 1

Life is not going to be as carefree and self-indulgent as it was before you had the responsibility of motherhood. But that doesn't mean you have to be a complete martyr. Even small steps can alleviate stress and break the cycle of overeating. Here are some suggestions for the first month.

CATCH-YOUR-BREATH EXERCISE: DEEP ABDOMINAL BREATHING

Deep abdominal breathing is a quick rejuvenator you can do with your baby beside you.

Lie down on a rug or towel and put your baby down next to you. Slowly exhale all the breath out of your mouth. Now put your hands on your abdomen. Inhale through your mouth and slowly fill up your abdomen with breath. As you inhale, fill up your lungs and feel your rib cage expand. Continue to inhale, filling up your chest. Hold the breath for 5 seconds, then exhale slowly through your nose.

Repeat the deep breathing sequence three or four times. Put your baby's hands on your tummy to keep her interested. She'll be amused by watching it go up and down with your breath.

As you become more adept at deep breathing, count to yourself: Inhale for 10 counts, hold for 5, exhale for 10. Think of inhaling energy and exhaling stress. When you've completed each exhalation, let your limbs relax into the ground—at least until the baby starts crawling or toddling away and you have to catch her.

DINNER DATE NIGHT

Since you're trying to eat early, you may be missing intimate, leisurely dinners with your partner. Set aside one day a week when you allow yourself to eat later, after the baby is (hopefully) asleep for the night. You can have a lovely, romantic evening without spending extra money on a restaurant or sitter. But you must make the effort to set aside a date night and keep the appointment, or it might never happen.

Select a dinner from the meal plans that you know your husband will enjoy. Prepare as much of it as you can beforehand.

Change out of your milk-splattered everyday clothes for the date, into an attractive outfit or silky lingerie. Light some candles and sip a glass of wine before dinner and see what happens . . . You might decide to go to bed before the meal and make love on an empty stomach. It's your choice, and your night to relax.

A LITTLE PAMPERING

You're so conscientious about making sure your baby is perfectly clean and powdered; soft hair smelling of baby shampoo; tiny fingernails trimmed. But are you taking any time for your own grooming? As a new mother you have every right to be as casual as you wish. Still, a little pampering is good for the soul.

Schedule one appointment of your choice this month: manicure, pedicure, hair cut, hair coloring, or facial. If you're on a budget, many nail salons offer lowered rates for services on Mondays, Tuesdays, and Wednesdays. For hair cuts and color, some salons offer discounts during student training nights or when they require models.

Ask for a cut that's low-maintenance, since your baby will probably short-circuit any lengthy styling sessions at home. Perhaps you stopped coloring your hair during your pregnancy and now you're ready for a change of color. Try something different to lift yourself out of the postpartum doldrums. You can be more alluring than ever with a fresh look and an adorable baby in tow.

MOMMY CARE MONTH 1 ACTION STEPS

1. Practice deep breathing to reduce stress and increase energy and well-being.

2. Savor a dinner date at home with your loved one.

3. Treat yourself to one professional beauty treatment—you deserve it!

PROGRESS EVALUATION FOR MONTH 1

Congratulations on completing your first month. Now it's time to step on the scale and compare the number to your preprogram weight. Hopefully, in addition to losing pounds, you notice your clothes are fitting better.

If you haven't lost weight as quickly as you expected or hoped, keep these points in mind:

- Rapid weight loss is mostly water loss. Numerous studies have shown that when you lose pounds slowly, you're more likely to keep them off.

- Consider where you are in your monthly cycle when you look at the scale. Many women are 3 to 7 pounds heavier before the onset of menstruation.

- Since muscle weighs more than fat, you can tone and trim without losing as many pounds as you'd expect.

Fitness is not a number on a scale, it's a state of being. So step back a minute to consider the other advantages of following the steps of the program. Check off which of these statements ring true:

☐ I'm more energetic.

☐ I'm less tense and irritable.

☐ I'm less moody.

☐ I have more patience with my baby.

☐ I have more interest in sex.

☐ I'm proud of myself.

☐ I feel stronger.

☐ My overall appearance is more attractive.

☐ I'm starting to look like my old self.

☐ Other people have commented that I look good.

Keep this checklist handy and refer to it when you need encouragement. Remind yourself frequently of all the benefits you're getting from the program, in addition to slimming down. Give yourself a pat on the back and enjoy the second month.

CHAPTER 7

MONTH 2:

Meal Plans, Workouts, and Mommy Care

In the first week of Month 2 you'll be preparing seven new meal plans, which you'll then repeat during the following three weeks of the month. Your fitness walks will become more challenging as you increase the intensity by measuring your target heart rate zone. You'll add the Supermom's Basic Strength-Training Routine to regain your prepregnancy tone—and perhaps get stronger than ever. And you'll start planning some special outings to expand your horizons and lift your spirits.

By this month, you should have a good understanding of the fundamental rules of safe weight loss and be somewhat accustomed to the smaller portions and low-fat food choices of the meal plans. But we all know there's a difference between eating because you're hungry and snacking for emotional reasons. If you're having trouble staying with the meal plans, step back and do a little analysis. Honestly assess the reason why you are eating, and see if you can substitute a healthier response than snacking. Some possibilities:

FEELING	WHAT YOU NEED
Tired	Lie down for a 20-minute nap.
	Or call it a night and go to bed, even if it's very early. Sometimes you have to sleep baby hours to get enough rest.
Anxious	Call someone you love or talk to your partner about your worries—but not in the kitchen.
	Or, exercise to reduce anxiety.
Bored	Throw yourself into a silly physical game with your baby.
	Or, when the baby's asleep, read a novel or biography that provides you with a few moments of escape.
Angry, resentful	Write down your grievances.
	Or write a letter to a person with whom you're angry. You don't have to show it to anyone; just get it out on paper.
	Or, put on music with a strong beat and jump around the room, wave your arms, dance, and shake it out.

SHOPPING CART LIST: MONTH 2

NOTE: You may already have some of these items left over from last month. Before shopping, check your supplies and cross off any items you already have in stock. At the beginning of weeks 2, 3, and 4 of this month, check the list to see what you need to replenish. Also add extra food for other family members as needed. Freeze breads to keep them fresh.

PRODUCE
Apple, 1
Banana, 1
Beans, kidney, 1 16-ounce can
Blueberries, fresh or frozen,
    1 pint
Broccoli florets, fresh or frozen,
    10 ounces
Cantaloupe, 1
Carrots, fresh baby, 1-pound
    bag
Celery, 1 bunch
Garlic bulb, 1
Grapes, seedless, 1 medium
    bunch
Lemons, 2
Mushrooms, fresh button,
    1 10-ounce package
Onions, 2-pound bag of
    yellow
Oranges, 2
Peas, green, 1 can or 1 package
    of frozen
Pears, 3
Pepper, green bell, 1
Potatoes, frozen hash brown
    patties, 1 package of 10
Potatoes, Idaho, 4
Raisins, 1 package of miniature
    boxes
Salad, prewashed blend of your
    choice, 2 bags
Shallots, 2
Spinach, 1 bag of fresh or
    1 package of frozen
Tangerine, 1
Tomatoes, 2 fresh

DAIRY
Butter, light, 1 8-ounce
    container (or 40%
    vegetable oil spread if
    preferred)
Cheese, cheddar low-fat,
    8 ounces
Cheese, mozzarella light
    shredded, 8 ounces
Cheese, grated Parmesan,
    8 ounces
Cottage cheese with pineapple,
    12 ounces
Cottage cheese, plain with small
    curds, 12 ounces
Eggs, 1 dozen

Egg product, Egg Beaters, 16
ounces
Milk, evaporated, 1 small can
Milk, nonfat (organic if you're
nursing), 1 gallon
Vanilla pudding, nonfat, 6-pack
of 4-ounce servings
Yogurt, nonfat flavor of choice,
3 8-ounce containers
Yogurt, frozen low-fat, flavor of
choice, 1 pint

MEAT/FISH
Bacon, nonfat turkey,
1 12-ounce package
Beef, top sirloin, 6 ounces (for
kebobs)
Fish fillets of choice, 4 4-ounce
fillets of orange roughy,
flounder, or cod
Ham lunch meat, nonfat 40%
ham/water sliced, 1 8-ounce
package
Lamb chops, 4 4-ounce center
loin
Tuna, 1 12-ounce can in water
Turkey breast, sliced, ¼ pound
Turkey, ground, 1 pound

GRAINS
Bread, bran with raisins, 1 loaf
Bread, Italian, 1 loaf
Bread, multigrain, 1 loaf
Bread, Pepperidge Farm garlic
bread (frozen)
Bread, pita, whole wheat, small,
1 package

Breadcrumbs, Italian
Breadsticks, Stella D'Oro,
1 package
Cereal, Barbara's Bakery
shredded wheat 97% fat-
free
Cereal bars, Nutrigrain Smart
Start strawberry, 1 box
Cereal, hot multigrain, 1 box of
instant packets
Cornmeal, white, 1 2-pound bag
Crackers, Snack Well's Classic
Golden Crackers, reduced
fat, 1 box
Crispbread, Weight Watchers
garlic, 1 package
English muffins, 1 package
Flour, white wheat, 1 2-pound
bag
Flour, whole wheat, 1 2-pound
bag
Pasta, whole wheat fettucine,
1 package
Rice, brown medium grain
instant, 1 6-ounce
package
Spaghetti, 1 16-ounce package

**SPICES, CONDIMENTS,
SAUCES, OIL**
Basil, ground
Canola oil spray
Celery salt
Cayenne pepper
Cumin seed
Dill weed, dried
Garlic powder

Italian seasoning
Ketchup
Lemon pepper seasoning
Mayonnaise, light
Mustard
Nutmeg, ground
Olive oil
Onion powder
Paprika
Parsley, dried
Pepper, black ground
Pickle relish, sweet
Rosemary, dried
Salad dressing, diet Italian
Salad dressing, low-fat
    Thousand Island
Salsa, mild, 1 jar
Salt
Spaghetti sauce, Prego chunky
    garden style, 1 27.5-ounce
    jar
Tomato sauce, 1 28-ounce can
Thyme, ground
Vegetable oil
Vegetable oil spread, 40% oil,
    8 ounces (or light butter)

MISC.
Almonds, sliced, 1 small package
Brownies, Weight Watchers
    frozen, 1 package
Burger mix, vegetarian
    meatless, 16 ounces
Corn chip snacks, Healthy
    Valley nonfat, 1 bag

Orange juice with added
    calcium, ½ gallon
Pizza, Weight Watchers lowfat
    frozen, 1 small pie
Popcorn, Gourmet microwave
    light butter-flavored
Pretzels, rods, 1 bag
Soup, Healthy Choice
    Minestrone, 1 10½-ounce
    can
Soup, Campbell's low salt with
    ribbon pasta, 1 10½-ounce
    can
Soup, Lipton's Spring
    Vegetable, 1 box
Vegetable juice, V-8, low-salt
    46 ounces
Walnuts or pecans, shelled, 1
    small bag
Wine, white table or cooking, 1
    small bottle
Wine, red table or cooking, 1
    small bottle

OPTIONAL
Additional breast-feeding
    bonus foods
Frozen dinners, low-fat and
    low-calorie
Fresh fruit for dessert
Seltzer water, flavored
Water, 3½–4½ gallons (if you
    have no filtering system)
Additional quantities of food
    for other family members

Month 2: Sunday

DAILY TOTALS, ALL FOODS

CALORIES	PROTEIN (G)	CARBS (G)	FAT (G)	SAT. FAT (G)	CHOL. (MG)	SODIUM (MG)	FIBER (G)
1534.40	110.64	212.97	30.53	11.25	85.02	3280.27	1702

BREAKFAST
Orange
Country Hash Browns and Egg Whites*, 1 serving
Multigrain bread, 1 slice
Cream cheese, nonfat, 1 ounce

MORNING MINI-MEAL
Cantaloupe, ¼
Cottage cheese, low-fat, ⅔ cup

LUNCH
Italian Grilled Cheese and Tomato Sandwich*
Pear
Nonfat milk, 1 cup

AFTERNOON MINI-MEAL
Popcorn, microwave, Gourmet, light butter-flavored, 4 cups

DINNER
Breaded Fish Fillets*, 1 serving
Salad dressing, diet Italian, 1 tablespoon
Breadsticks, Stella D'Oro, 2

Nonfat milk, 1 cup
Brownie, frozen, Weight Watchers, 1

Substitute fresh fruit for dessert if desired. Add breast-feeding bonus foods (pages 60–62) as needed—see Chapter 4.

*See Chapter 9 for recipes.

Month 2: Monday

DAILY TOTALS, ALL FOODS

CALORIES	PROTEIN (G)	CARBS (G)	FAT (G)	SAT. FAT (G)	CHOL. (MG)	SODIUM (MG)	FIBER (G)
1536.29	85.93	279.13	19.49	4.44	22.12	2632.35	21.94

BREAKFAST
Multigrain hot cereal, instant, 1 packet
Banana, ½

MORNING MINI-MEAL
Yogurt, nonfat, any flavor, 8 ounces

LUNCH
Multigrain bread, 1 slice
Cheddar cheese, low-fat, 1 slice
Salad dressing, low-fat Thousand Island, 1 tablespoon
Spinach, raw, 1 cup
Nonfat milk, 1 cup

AFTERNOON MINI-MEAL
Apple

DINNER

Veggie Chili*, 1 serving

Tossed salad, 1½ cups

Salad dressing, diet Italian, 1½ tablespoons

Garlic crispbread, Weight Watchers, 2 crackers

Brownie, Weight Watchers, 1

Nonfat milk, 1 cup

Substitute fresh fruit for dessert if desired. Add breast-feeding bonus foods (pages 60–62) as needed—see Chapter 4.

*See Chapter 9 for recipes.

Month 2: Tuesday

DAILY TOTALS, ALL FOODS

CALORIES	PROTEIN (G)	CARBS (G)	FAT (G)	SAT. FAT (G)	CHOL. (MG)	SODIUM (MG)	FIBER (G)
1636.38	96.18	212.07	45.80	13.53	339.06	2244.70	19.87

BREAKFAST

1 Scrambled egg, cooked with canola oil spray

Bran bread with raisins, 1 slice

Light butter or 40% vegetable oil spread, 1 tablespoon

Nonfat milk, 1 cup

MORNING MINI-MEAL

Yogurt, nonfat, any flavor, 8 ounces

LUNCH

Italian Grilled Cheese and Tomato Sandwich*

Pear

Nonfat milk, 1 cup

AFTERNOON MINI-MEAL
Cereal bar, Nutrigrain Smart Start strawberry

DINNER
Lamb Chops with Shallots and Red Wine*, 1 serving
Green peas, canned or frozen, ½ cup
Potato, baked, 1 medium
Light butter or 40% vegetable oil spread for potato, 1 tablespoon
Nonfat milk, 1 cup
Vanilla pudding, nonfat

Substitute fresh fruit for dessert if desired. Add breast-feeding bonus foods (pages 60–62) as needed—see Chapter 4.

*See Chapter 9 for recipes.

Month 2: Wednesday

DAILY TOTALS, ALL FOODS

CALORIES	PROTEIN (G)	CARBS (G)	FAT (G)	SAT. FAT (G)	CHOL. (MG)	SODIUM (MG)	FIBER (G)
1536.59	99.34	235.16	28.62	10.55	60.14	3158.46	17.36

BREAKFAST
Salsa Breakfast Scramble*, 1 serving
Vegetable juice, V-8, low-salt, 1 cup

MORNING MINI-MEAL
Orange
Cheddar cheese, 1 ounce
Nonfat milk, 1 cup

LUNCH
Turkey Sandwich*
Minestrone soup, Healthy Choice, 1 cup

AFTERNOON MINI-MEAL
Celery, 2 small stalks
Low-fat Thousand Island dressing, 1 tablespoon
Crispbread, Weight Watchers garlic, 2 crackers

DINNER
Low-fat Fettucine Alfredo*, 1 serving
Tossed salad, 1½ cups
Salad dressing, diet Italian, 1 tablespoon
Nonfat milk, 1 cup
Cantaloupe, ¼
Yogurt, nonfat, any flavor, 8 ounces

Add breast-feeding bonus foods (pages 60–62) as needed—see Chapter 4.

*See Chapter 9 for recipes.

Month 2: Thursday

DAILY TOTALS, ALL FOODS

CALORIES	PROTEIN (G)	CARBS (G)	FAT (G)	SAT. FAT (G)	CHOL. (MG)	SODIUM (MG)	FIBER (G)
1517.45	83.24	234.08	34.53	7.27	95.49	2223.48	13.97

BREAKFAST
Multigrain hot cereal, instant, 1 packet
Banana, ½ medium
Orange juice, 1 cup

MORNING MINI-MEAL
Cereal bar, Nutrigrain Smart Start strawberry

LUNCH

Cottage cheese, low-fat, with pineapple, ½ cup

Blueberries, 1 cup, frozen thawed or fresh

Bran bread with raisins, 1 slice

Light butter or 40% vegetable oil spread, 1 tablespoon

Nonfat milk, 1 cup

AFTERNOON MINI-MEAL

Pretzels, 1 ounce

DINNER

Steak and Vegetable Kabobs *

Tossed salad, 1½ cups

Salad dressing, low-fat Thousand Island, 1 tablespoon

Nonfat milk, 1 cup

Chocolate chip cookie, lowfat Snackwell's, 1

Substitute fresh fruit for dessert if desired. Add breast-feeding bonus foods (pages 60–62) as needed—see Chapter 4.

*See Chapter 9 for recipes.

Month 2: Friday

DAILY TOTALS, ALL FOODS

CALORIES	PROTEIN (G)	CARBS (G)	FAT (G)	SAT. FAT (G)	CHOL. (MG)	SODIUM (MG)	FIBER (G)
1513.16	79.15	249.55	29.75	5.46	99.81	2532.59	18.84

BREAKFAST

Shredded wheat cereal, Barbara's Bakery, 2 biscuits

Nonfat milk, 1 cup

Raisins, 1 miniature box

Orange juice, 1 cup

MORNING MINI-MEAL
Pear
SnackWell's Classic Golden Crackers, reduced fat, 6

LUNCH
Chicken soup, Campbell's with ribbon pasta, 1 cup
Make a sandwich with:
Bacon, turkey, 80% fat-free, 1 slice cooked with canola oil spray
Low-fat Cheddar cheese, 1 ounce slice
Tomato, 1 slice
Multigrain bread, 2 slices
Nonfat milk, 1 cup

AFTERNOON MINI-MEAL
Grapes, 10
Corn chip snack, nonfat Healthy Valley, 1 ounce

DINNER
Mom's Turkey Meatloaf*, 1 serving
Broccoli florets, fresh or frozen, 3.3 ounces
Tossed salad, 1½ cup
Salad dressing, low-fat Thousand Island, 1 tablespoon
Italian bread, 1 slice
Light butter or 40% vegetable oil spread
Yogurt, frozen, low-fat, 1 cup

Add breast-feeding bonus foods (pages 60–62) as needed—see Chapter 4.
*See Chapter 9 for recipes.

Month 2: Saturday

CALORIES	PROTEIN (G)	CARBS (G)	FAT (G)	SAT. FAT (G)	CHOL. (MG)	SODIUM (MG)	FIBER (G)
1527.25	99.95	204.38	38.06	9.90	316.07	3238.04	14.64

BREAKFAST

1 Scrambled egg, cooked with canola oil spray

Multigrain bread, 1 slice toasted

Cream cheese, nonfat, 2 tablespoons

Nonfat milk, 1 cup

MORNING MINI-MEAL

Vegetable juice, V-8 low-salt, 1 cup

SnackWell's Classic Golden Crackers, reduced fat, 12

LUNCH

Pizza, low-fat, Weight Watchers Deluxe Combination, 1 small pie

Tangerine

Carrots, 4 baby

Nonfat milk, 1 cup

AFTERNOON MINI-MEAL

Popcorn, Gourmet microwave light butter-flavored, 4 cups

DINNER

Spaghetti and Modern Meatballs*, 1 serving

Garlic bread, frozen, Pepperidge Farm, 1 slice

Nonfat milk, 1 cup

Vanilla pudding, nonfat, 1 serving

Substitute fresh fruit for dessert if desired. Add breast-feeding bonus foods (pages 60–62) as needed—see Chapter 4.

*See Chapter 9 for recipes.

MOTHER'S SLIMMING REMINDERS

- *Drink plenty of fluids*: Eight glasses of water per day; ten glasses of water if you're nursing. For a change of pace, try adding a twist of lemon or lime to your ice water.

- *Eat early*. Finish dinner by 6:30 P.M., except on one special dinner-date night each week. Save your dessert for 8:00 if you know you'll be craving a snack.

- *Whenever possible, sit down and eat slowly*, to allow time to feel satisfied. Sitting is not always an option when you have a baby. But if you have a chance to eat during baby's nap time or when she is mellow, slow down and enjoy your meal.

WORKABLE WORKOUTS FOR MONTH 2

This month, you'll be continuing with your fitness walks. The goal is to walk more often, faster, and further. Participate in fitness walking or your substitute aerobic exercise at least three times a week, for 30 to 45 minutes each session. Start off at a slower pace for the first 5 to 10 minutes to warm up, then increase the intensity.

YOUR TARGET HEART RATE ZONE

At this point, you may be ready to make your workout a little more scientific. If you're so inclined, you can figure out your target heart rate (THR) zone and use it as a tool for measuring the intensity of your aerobic workout and its cardiovascular benefits.

The traditional time to calculate your heart rate is when you first wake up, before getting out of bed. But if you've been awakened by a crying baby, this may not be the best moment to get a resting reading. Select a time when you're relaxed and calm.

With your index and middle fingers, locate your pulse on the inside of your wrist on the thumb side (with palm up), or on the side of your throat (under your jawline). Using a watch or a clock with a second hand, count the number of beats in your pulse in ten seconds. Then multiply this number by 6 to arrive at your resting heart rate (RHR). This figure will normally be in the range of sixty to eighty beats per minute—in other words, an RHR of 60 to 80.

Next, use the Karvonen formula to determine your THR zone. Unless you're a math wizard you'll need a piece of scratch paper. The following example is for a thirty-year-old woman with a RHR of 70.

Start with the standard figure of 220:	220
Subtract your age:	−30
Your maximum heart rate is:	190
Subtract your resting heart rate:	−70
Your heart rate reserve is:	120
Multiply by 60%:	×.60
	72
Add your RHR:	+70
	142
Now, multiply your heart rate reserve by 80%:	120
	×.80
	96
Add your RHR:	+70
	166

The two highlighted figures are the target heart rate (THR) zone. For the woman in this example, the THR zone is 142 to 166 beats per minutes, which is 60 to 80 percent of maximum heart rate.

If you've made it through this calculation without being distracted by your baby, be assured that you won't have to do it again. Once you know your THR zone, all you need to do is tap into your pulse about 10 minutes into your fitness walk or alternative aerobic exercise to see if you're in the right range of intensity. Count your pulse rate for 10 seconds, then multiply by six. If your pulse is above the higher number of your THR zone, slow down. If it's slower than the lower number of your THR zone, step up the pace.

If you can't manage to count your pulse while walking with the stroller (which can be tricky), there are other ways to measure the intensity of your pace. These other methods are more subjective, but still useful. One approach is to categorize how hard you perceive you are working your heart, using these adjectives:

- Very light

- Fairly light

- Somewhat hard

- Hard

- Very hard

- Very, very hard

By the second month of the program (provided you don't have any special health concerns), you should be working out in the "somewhat hard" to "hard" range.

Another barometer: When you are fitness walking, your heart should be beating faster than normal (but not to the point of feeling breathless or dizzy). Breaking into a light sweat on a warm day is also a good indicator that the intensity is sufficient.

Then again, if you really want to obtain accuracy, sporting goods stores offer a wide range of devices to measure heartbeat, intensity, mileage, etc.

INDOOR AEROBIC ALTERNATIVE: EXERCISE MACHINES

One choice for indoor days is a treadmill or exercise bike, if you have space for one now that your home is filled with baby gear. Treadmills and exercise bicycles come in many styles, from basic to high-tech contraptions that measure every movement. It's wise to start with a basic model until you're sure you will use it. Yard sales are littered with discarded exercise equipment from people with good intentions.

Plant the treadmill or exercise bicycle near a TV or a CD player, since pacing or peddling to nowhere can be quite tedious without accompaniment. Upbeat music can also help you stay motivated. Try to keep going for thirty minutes.

To keep an older baby occupied during treadmill time, you may have to nestle him somewhere comfortable and turn on his favorite TV show. (Don't feel guilty; he'll still grow up to be a genius.) Another idea is to have a portable playpen situated near the machine and hope that your baby will stay content with some toys. But more likely he'll be clamoring to get out and climb on the treadmill with you—*not* a safe idea for a young child.

> **REMINDER:** Whether you walk outside, use an exercise machine indoors, or do the freelance dance, start off at a moderate pace to warm up, then increase the intensity after 5 or 10 minutes. Afterward, do the cool-down stretches on pages 118–20.

STRENGTH TRAINING

Right now you can probably carry your darling little baby in your arms almost effortlessly, but someday soon he'll be a 30-pound toddler who needs to be corralled. It's best to build up your strength now, before he gets any bigger!

Besides the obvious advantages of being a strong mother, strength training will help you achieve these desirable results:

- Flatter stomach

- Smaller waist

- Higher, firmer breasts

- Firmer thighs

- Better posture (which alone can make you look 5 to 10 pounds thinner).

In addition, strength-training workouts increase your metabolic rate, so you burn more calories during *all* your activities, from sleeping to walking. It takes more calories to maintain lean muscle than it does to maintain fat. By increasing the percentage of muscle versus fat, you automatically increase the number of calories your body burns throughout the day. That's why strength training is considered an integral part of a weight-loss/fitness program.

Strength training can also reduce a susceptibility to back pain and injury. This is an important consideration since child-care requires a great deal of bending down and scrunching your spine.

Don't confuse strength training with weight lifting and worry about developing muscles that are too big for your taste. Most strength-training routines use moderately light hand-held weights, along with your own body weight, to tone and strengthen without bulking up.

There are several ways to approach strength training:

- A videotape (see suggestions on pages 171–74)

- A personal trainer, if you have the time and money for this wonderful luxury

- A class at a gym that provides baby-sitting (once your baby is old enough). Many classes combine aerobic exercise and strength training.

You can also start with the Supermom's Basic Strength-Training Routine, which follows. Try this set of exercises after your aerobic walk, or instead of walking on rainy days. Perform it two or three times a week and you'll begin to feel firmer and more power-ful. All you need to get started is a set of 3-to-5-pound weights, an exercise mat or rug, and flexible clothing. Start with the 3-pound weights if you're new to strength training; use 5-pound weights if you've had experience with this kind of exercise.

SUPERMOM'S BASIC STRENGTH-TRAINING ROUTINE

WARM-UP

Make sure your baby is fed and diapered. Settle her down somewhere comfortably where she can watch you.

Standing Stretch

Stand with your feet hip-width apart. Lift your arms to the side and then up. Alternate stretching your right arm up and then your left arm up, 4 times on each side. Concentrate on stretching the whole side of your body as you lift your arm. Lower your arms when you're finished.

Head and Neck Warm-up

Slowly turn your head right and left, 4 times to each side. Then slowly roll your head around to the right 4 times and the left 4 times. Don't let your neck drop all the way to the back; keep it a little lifted.

Shoulder Stretch

Shrug your shoulders up and down, 4 times each. Press your shoulders back and forward, 4 times each. Roll your shoulders to the back 4 times; to the front 4 times. Place your hands on your shoulders. Circle your elbows so that they touch in the front, then reach toward the back; 4 circles in each direction.

Twist

Lift your arms to the side. Gently twist your upper body and torso from side to side 8 times, keeping your hips facing front. Twist to each side 8 times.

Lower Body Warm-up (Plié)

Stand with your legs hip-width apart and your feet turned out, arms to the side. Slowly bend your knees. Then straighten your legs and come up onto the balls of your feet (or "half-toe," as they say in the dance world). Repeat this sequence 8 times.

STRENGTH-BUILDING EXERCISES

Squats

BENEFITS: thighs and buttocks

Hold a 3–5 pound weight in each hand. Stand with your feet a little wider than hip-width, arms down, elbows slightly bent. Keep your back straight and your abdominal muscles firm as you bend your knees and sit back into a squat. Keep your buttocks and abs tight as you straighten your legs to the starting position. Do 1 set of 20 repetitions for the first few sessions. When you feel ready, do 2 sets each time.

HINTS:

- If you find these difficult, begin without weights. Hold onto a piece of furniture for support.

- Never go lower than a 90-degree angle in a squat.

- If you have knee problems or stiffness, begin with a partial squat, keeping your knees at a 45-degree angle.

- If your baby is restless, hold her in your arms in front of your body instead of holding weights as you perform the squats.

Rows

BENEFITS: rhomboids (midback), latissimus dorsi (back), biceps (front of arms)

Stand with your feet shoulder-width apart and knees slightly bent. Hold your 3–5 pound weight in each hand. Tighten your abdominal muscles and keep your back flat as you bend slightly forward from your hips. Keep your elbows bent and your arms close to your body. Then move your elbows back in a rowing motion. Slowly return to the starting position. Do 1 set of 20–25 rows.

HINTS:

- Add more rows and additional weight as you get stronger. This exercise strengthens your back, which will help your posture and enhance the appearance of your bust.

- Sing "Row, row, row your boat" to your baby to amuse her while doing rows.

Bent-Knee Push-ups

BENEFITS: pectorals (chest), triceps (back of arms)

Start with your weight resting on straight arms and bent knees, your face toward the floor and your back straight. Cross your feet and hold them slightly off the ground. Keep your back straight as you use your arm strength to lower your weight to the floor, bending at the elbows. Then push up, again keeping your back straight. Do 2 sets of 10.

HINTS:

- Inhale as you lower your body, exhale as you push up.

- If you already have a lot of upper-body strength, you can start with the classic push-ups. These are done with your weight on your hands and feet, and your entire body straight.

- Put your baby on her tummy on the floor next to you as you do push-ups. She'll probably mimic you with her own little push-up, one of the first "exercises" babies can do.

Ab Crunches

BENEFITS: abdominals

Lie on your back on a padded surface. Bend your knees and place your feet flat on the floor. Press your lower back into the floor so there is no arch. Rest your head in your hands. Tighten your abdominals muscles and slowly lift your shoulders off the floor as you exhale. Slowly lower your upper body back to the floor as you inhale. Start with 1 set of 20 crunches. The second week do 2 sets each session.

HINTS:

- Don't tighten your neck or shoulders. Concentrate on using your abdominal muscles to move your body up and down.

- Rub your neck afterward to make sure there's no tension.

- Keep your lower back pressed into the floor and keep breathing.

- Put your baby alongside you on the floor. Turn crunches into a game by making a funny noise as you exhale. One of the wonderful qualities of babies is that they find almost anything you do amusing!

Straddle stretch: Sit on the floor with your legs straight and feet wide apart. Put your baby between your legs. Keeping your torso fairly straight, stretch forward and hug. You should feel a gentle stretch in your hamstrings. Then stretch your left arm to the right leg, feeling the stretch in your waist. Hold for 10 seconds, then bring your arms center. Repeat to the other side. Repeat the whole sequence.

Cobra: Lie down on your stomach. Bend your elbows and place your hands, palms flat on the floor, 5 inches out from your shoulders. Slowly inhale and lift your head, shoulders, and upper back. Be gentle and don't hyperextend backward. Keep your hip bones on the floor. Hold for 10 seconds, then roll down. Repeat. An older baby will enjoy climbing on your back as you do this stretch.

If you have time, you can also do the cool-down stretches on pages 118–20.

WORKABLE WORKOUT MONTH 2 ACTION STEPS

1. Continue to walk with your baby, 30 to 45 minutes, three times a week or more. Walk at a brisk pace and include some hills.

2. Do an alternative aerobic workout on indoor days.

3. Do the cool-down stretches after your fitness walk or aerobic exercise.

4. Do strength-training exercises twice a week, stretching before and afterward.

MOMMY CARE

Quite often, new mothers are so in love with their babies that they abandon all their other interests. While this is natural and fulfilling for the first few months, by the time your baby is three or four months old you need a change of pace or you'll go stir-crazy. It will help your emotional health in the long run to get in the habit of planning an occasional outing for yourself. Just one half-day or evening twice a month can make a difference and keep your world from closing in.

What are some of the activities you enjoyed doing before you had a baby and haven't had time for since? Some possibilities:

- Going to the movies

- Going out to dinner

- Visiting a museum

- Shopping with a girlfriend

- Hearing live music

- Going out to dance and "party"

- Having a weekend away

- Hiking or biking

This month, pick two of these activities or whatever else it is that you miss doing most. Figure out when a family member or a baby-sitter will be available and make two dates to indulge in your favorite activities. Book your relative or baby-sitter now, even if the date is two weeks ahead. Mark down the dates on your calendar.

Each month, plan one or two outings that do not revolve around your baby. These excursions keep your spirits up and your outlook fresh.

HYDROTHERAPY

Hydrotherapy—the therapeutic use of water—is a divine treat for mothers, who are always lifting, twisting, and otherwise contorting themselves. Water is soothing, sensual, and invigorating.

Outdoor spas are one of the ultimate pleasures. If you have an opportunity to install one on your property, it's a wonderful luxury. Yes, they are expensive, but ultimately a good value when compared to spending money on vacations (especially since traveling with a baby can be less than relaxing).

Another choice is to find a location that has an indoor or outdoor hot tub you can use. This might be a "Y," health club, or hotel. Don't forget to do your exercise *before* going in the whirlpool; afterward you'll be too mellow to move.

A word of caution: Spas and hot tubs, whether freestanding or in the bathtub, are not safe or appropriate for babies. This is an adults-only pleasure. If you have an outdoor spa that you keep filled with water, you must take appropriate precautions about covering it and enclosing it in a fence.

If a full-size outdoor spa is not a possibility at this point, you may be able to purchase a bathtub with hydrotherapy features. Or, for under $100, you can buy a whirlpool attachment that sits in your bathtub and creates bubbles and jets of soothing water. Another option is a shower massage unit. How soothing that pulsing water feels on neck and shoulder muscles that are strained from bending over baby and shouldering a diaper bag.

You can even turn an ordinary bath into a retreat. Scented candles for the bath are available with different fragrances to evoke various moods. (For safety's sake, place them far away from a crawling baby's reach and extinguish them as soon as you're done.) Bath oils are a pleasant, aromatic touch. You can listen to some relaxing music while you're in the tub. Drape a hot washcloth over your neck or shoulders to release those hard-working mommy muscles.

After the bath, cuddle up in a warm terrycloth robe and spa slippers. Smooth some herbal lotion over your skin to moisturize. You'll feel smooth and smell delicious.

TOP TEN STRESS-REDUCERS FOR MOMS AT HOME

1. Nap once during the day for at least 20 minutes while your baby's napping.

2. Play music that you enjoy frequently throughout the day.

3. Try not to watch too many talk shows or news shows during the day; it's not positive input for you or your baby.

4. Play classical music or other relaxing music while you're doing household chores or babycare.

5. Schedule visits with other moms as often as possible. Even if the babies are too young to play, it's good for *your* mental health to talk to another adult.

6. Spend as much time as possible outside during the nice weather. If you don't have a yard or patio, find a nice

park, playground, church ground, or other area where you can sit.

7. Sing to your baby throughout the day. It's great for your soul and for his.

8. Don't try to be a perfect housekeeper. If you have the budget, bring in a cleaning person at least once every two weeks. The fact that you're home doesn't mean you have time to do everything.

9. Don't blame yourself if your baby's not happy all the time. He may be teething, or have a tummy ache or any number of little gripes he can't express yet. Don't overreact; these moods and stages pass quickly.

10. When you feel overwhelmed, remember that it gets easier every year. The first year is the hardest, the second year is the second hardest, and by the time your baby is three it gets easy.

BEATING THE BACK-TO-WORK BLUES

If you have a full-time career, you may have even less opportunity than stay-at-home moms to catch up on sleep, see friends, and take time for personal nourishment. And so, the tendency to turn to comfort foods to "treat" yourself and alleviate stress is a danger.

There are no easy answers to the many issues involved in balancing motherhood and a career. It's a gradual, ever-changing process in which you'll need the support of your co-workers, family, and friends. Meanwhile, a few of the following simple steps can help reduce your stress level.

TOP TEN STRESS-REDUCERS FOR MOMS WHO WORK OUTSIDE THE HOME

1. Commute by bus or train so that your commuting time can become "downtime."

2. Read a novel on the train or bus instead of a newspaper (since most news is bad news and is hardly relaxing).

3. Or, use your bus/train time as a brief respite where you drift between dozing and dreaming, allowed to do nothing for the only time all day.

4. If you drive to work, listen to books on tape or quality CDs in the car. Consider carpooling so you don't have to deal with traffic every day.

5. Exercise at least twice a week at lunchtime. Keep sneakers in your desk for a brisk fitness walk. Or look into the feasibility of going to a gym or workout class.

6. See non-work friends at lunchtime once a week if possible. If you always eat with colleagues, conversation tends to be about work and it's less of a break. It can also be relaxing to eat lunch alone.

7. Pack your lunch and snacks with meals from the HELP for Moms Menu the night before to avoid a morning crunch.

8. If you can possibly afford it, have your house cleaned professionally once every two weeks. This will take one task off your plate.

9. Don't project your feelings onto your baby. You may miss him more than he misses you at this stage. Babies have a great

capacity for living in the moment. If he is with a kind caregiver, he is probably happy, not pining away for you all day.

10. Remember that being a working mother is not unnatural or inherently wrong. In many cultures and periods throughout history, mothers have worked while their babies were cared for by other family members or neighbors. Home care or a daycare center with an attentive, affectionate staff can be a modern extension of this type of arrangement.

MOMMY CARE MONTH 2 ACTION STEPS

1. Make a date for at least one special activity/outing this month. Line up your baby-sitter and put it on your calendar.

2. Indulge in some form of hydrotherapy.

3. Use the Top Ten Stress Reducers to lighten your load.

PROGRESS EVALUATION FOR MONTH 2

After two months of exercise, you should be seeing some encouraging toning effects. In addition to "weighing in," measure your waist and hips. Then compare these measurements with your Preprogram Record.

Also do a mirror check. You'll probably notice improved posture and a more lifted look to your body. You're feeling more comfortable in your body, confident, and ready for the final stage of the program.

CHAPTER 8

MONTH 3:

Meal Plans, Workouts, and Mommy Care

Month 3 is the momentum month. You will step up the pace of your aerobic workouts and increase the repetitions of the strength-building exercises. Combined with the low-fat diet, this should produce additional weight loss and toning. It may be hard to maintain your discipline, but after two months of results you know it's worth it. Keep going—the third month is the charm!

The HELP Rules for Weight Loss should be second nature by now:

- *Eat early*. Finish by 6:30 P.M. most nights, except for breast-feeding bonus foods or a saved dessert at 8 P.M.

- *Eat less, but more frequently*. As the meal plans prescribe, divide your food consumption into five mini-meals a day. Have your first meal no more than a half hour after you wake up, so you don't start the day hungry. Space each meal out every two to three hours.

- *Eat low-fat foods*, such as those in the meal plans.

- *Drink lots of water*. Eight glasses per day, ten glasses per day if you're breast-feeding. Drink water with any meals that don't specify another drink. (NOTE: You can have up to two cups of coffee or tea a day and up to two alcoholic drinks a week without any detriment to the diet. If you're nursing, make your own informed decisions about alcohol and caffeine.)

NOTE: You may already have some of these items left over from last month. Before shopping, check your supplies and cross off any items you already have in stock. At the beginning of weeks 2, 3, and 4 of this month, check the list to see what you need to replenish. Also add extra food for other family members as needed. Freeze breads to keep them fresh.

PRODUCE
Apples, 3
Asparagus spears, 20 fresh
    spears or 1 8-ounce pack-
    age of frozen
Banana, 1
Blueberries, fresh or frozen,
    1 pint
Broccoli, fresh, 1 small bunch
Broccoli florets, fresh or frozen,
    1 10-ounce package
Carrots, fresh baby, 1-pound bag
Celery, 1 bunch
Corn on the cob, fresh or
    frozen, 4 ears
Garlic, 1 bulb
Grapefruit, 1
Grapes, seedless, 1 medium
    bunch
Lemons, 2
Limes, 2
Mushrooms, fresh button,
    1 10-ounce package
Mushrooms, fresh shiitake,
    8 ounces
Onion, 1 white

Onions, green, 1 bunch
Oranges, 3
Peach, 1
Peppers, green bell, 4
Plum, 1
Potatoes, frozen hash brown
    patties, 1 package of 10
Salad, prewashed blend of your
    choice, 1 bag
Strawberries, fresh or frozen,
    10 ounces
Tangerine, 1
Tomatoes, 2 large

DAIRY
Butter, light, 1 8-ounce con-
    tainer (or 40% vegetable
    oil spread if preferred)
Cheese, cheddar low-fat,
    8 ounces
Cheese, grated Parmesan,
    8 ounces
Chocolate pudding, nonfat,
    6 4-ounce servings
Cottage cheese with pineapple,
    12 ounces

Cream cheese, light, 8 ounces
Eggs, 1 dozen
Egg product, Egg Beaters,
    16 ounces
Milk, light buttermilk, 1 quart
Milk, 2%, 1 quart
Milk, nonfat (organic if you're
    nursing), 1 gallon
Yogurt, low-fat flavor of choice,
    1 8-ounce containers
Yogurt, frozen low-fat, flavor of
    choice, 1 pint

MEAT/FISH
Beef bottom round, trimmed to
    ¼-inch fat and cut into
    strips, 1 pound
Crabmeat, 2 6-ounce cans
Tuna, 1 12-ounce can in water
Tuna steak, fresh yellowfin, cut
    into 4 portions
Turkey, ground, 1 pound
Veal leg, top round sliced scal-
    lopini style, 1 pound

GRAINS
Bread, bran with raisins, 1 loaf
Bread, Italian, 1 loaf
Bread, multigrain, 1 loaf
Bread, Pepperidge Farm dinner
    rolls
Bread, white, low-salt, 1 loaf,
Bread, pita, whole wheat, small,
    package of 4
Breadcrumbs, Italian
Cereal, Cheerios

Cereal, hot multigrain, 1 box of
    instant packets
Cereal, Post 100% Bran
Couscous, 1 12-ounce box
Cornmeal, white, 1 2-pound
    bag
Crackers, Snack Well's Classic
    Golden Crackers, reduced
    fat, 1 box
English muffins, 1 package of 4
Noodles, Japanese Udon,
    1 7-ounce package
Noodles, No-yolk egg, 12
    ounces
Oatmeal, wholegrain instant, 16
    ounces
Tortillas, 4 low-fat burrito-
    sized, 1 package

**SPICES, CONDIMENTS,
SAUCES, OIL**
Basil, ground
Butter substitute, Butter Bud
    Sprinkles, 1 box of
    packets
Canola oil
Canola oil spray
Capers, small jar
Celery salt
Cinnamon, ground
Garlic, ground
Ginger, ground
Ketchup
Mayonnaise, light
Mustard
Olive oil, extra virgin

Paprika
Peanut butter, chunky,
    1 8-ounce jar
Pepper, black ground
Pickle relish, sweet
Preserves, blueberry
Rosemary, dried
Salad dressing, diet French
Salad dressing, low-fat Thou-
    sand Island
Salsa, mild, 1 small jar
Salt
Soy sauce, low sodium teriyaki,
    light
Sugar, brown, 1 1-pound bag
Vanilla extract
Vegetable oil spread, 40% oil,
    8 ounces (or light butter)
Vinegar, red wine
Worcestershire sauce

MISC.
Brownies, Weight Watchers
    frozen, 1 package
Champagne, 1 bottle
Cookies, Health Valley granola,
    1 box
Orange juice with added
    calcium, ½ gallon
Pancake mix, light
Pancake syrup, light
Pizza, Healthy Choice French
    Bread Cheese, 1 pie

Popcorn, Gourmet microwave
    light butter-flavored
Sorbet, Dole nonfat strawberry,
    1 pint
Soup, Progresso beef barley,
    1 15-ounce can
Soup, Swanson 99% fat-free
    chicken broth, 1 32-ounce
    can or carton
Soup, Healthy Choice Mine-
    strone, 1 15-ounce can
Soup, Healthy Choice Tomato
    Garden, 1 15-ounce can
Tortilla Chips, Guiltless
    Gourmet baked, 1 7-ounce
    package
Vegetable juice, V-8 low-salt,
    1 46-ounce bottle
Whipped topping, light,
    1 8-ounce container
Wine, white cooking

OPTIONAL
Additional breast-feeding
    bonus foods
Seltzer water, flavored
Frozen dinners, low-fat and
    low-calorie
Fresh fruit for dessert
Water, 3½–4½ gallons (if you
    have no filtering system)
Additional quantities of food
    for other family members

MEAL PLANS

Month 3: Sunday

DAILY TOTALS, ALL FOODS

CALORIES	PROTEIN (G)	CARBS (G)	FAT (G)	SAT. FAT (G)	CHOL. (MG)	SODIUM (MG)	FIBER (G)
1606.65	85.95	263.20	27.46	8.46	59.08	1915.42	13.74

BREAKFAST

French Toast*, 1 serving

Strawberries, fresh or frozen and thawed, ½ cup

Nonfat milk, 1 cup

MORNING MINI-MEAL

Orange

Cottage cheese, low-fat with pineapple, ½ cup

LUNCH

French Bread Cheese Pizza, Healthy Choice, 5.6 oz

Nonfat milk, 1 cup

AFTERNOON MINI-MEAL

Apple

DINNER

Couscous-Stuffed Peppers*, 1 serving

Tossed salad, 1½ cups

Salad dressing, low-fat Thousand Island, 1 tablespoon

Dinner roll, Pepperidge Farm Classic Country Style, 1

Light butter or 40% vegetable oil spread, 1 tablespoon

Chocolate pudding snack, nonfat

Substitute fresh fruit for dessert if desired. Add breast-feeding bonus foods (pages 60–62) as needed—see Chapter 4.

*See Chapter 9 for recipes.

Month 3: Monday

CALORIES	PROTEIN (G)	CARBS (G)	FAT (G)	SAT. FAT (G)	CHOL. (MG)	SODIUM (MG)	FIBER (G)
1577.96	100.51	220.56	35.02	9.40	156.62	2937.30	14.87

BREAKFAST
Multigrain hot cereal, instant, ¾ cup
Banana, ½ medium

MORNING MINI-MEAL
Bran bread with raisins, 1 slice
Cream cheese, nonfat, 1 ounce

LUNCH
Tomato Garden Soup, Healthy Choice, 1 cup
Make a sandwich with:
Multigrain bread, 2 slices
Cheddar cheese, 1 ounce, sliced
Light mayonnaise, 1 tablespoon

AFTERNOON MINI-MEAL
Yogurt, low-fat, 8 ounces

DINNER
Grilled Thai Ginger Tuna Steak*, 1 serving
Corn on the cob, 1 ear
Light butter or 40% vegetable oil spread, ½ tablespoon
Brownie, Weight Watchers, 1

Substitute fresh fruit for dessert if desired. Add breast-feeding bonus foods (pages 60–62) as needed—see Chapter 4.

*See Chapter 9 for recipes.

Month 3: Tuesday

CALORIES	PROTEIN (G)	CARBS (G)	FAT (G)	SAT. FAT (G)	CHOL. (MG)	SODIUM (MG)	FIBER (G)
1603.40	81.80	214.37	59.10	13.77	147.20	2881.68	36.95

BREAKFAST
Bran cereal, Post 100% Bran, 1 cup
Milk, nonfat, 1 cup
Blueberries, fresh or frozen and thawed, ½ cup

MORNING MINI-MEAL
Apple, cut into 8 slices
Peanut butter, chunky, 2 tablespoons, spread on apple

LUNCH
Italian Grilled Cheese and Tomato Sandwich*
Milk, nonfat, 1 cup

AFTERNOON MINI-MEAL
Popcorn, Gourmet microwave light butter-flavored, 3 cups
Tangerine

DINNER
Veal Scallopini with Lemon-Caper Sauce*, 1 serving
Broccoli florets, frozen, and cooked according to package, 1
    serving (3 ounces)
Italian bread, 1 slice
Light butter or 40% vegetable oil spread, 1 tablespoon
Sorbet, Dole nonfat strawberry, ½ cup

Add bread-feeding bonus foods (pages 60–62) as needed—see Chapter 4.
*See Chapter 9 for recipes.

Month 3: Wednesday

CALORIES	PROTEIN (G)	CARBS (G)	FAT (G)	SAT. FAT (G)	CHOL. (MG)	SODIUM (MG)	FIBER (G)
1501.78	104.04	213.27	30.33	11.05	193.48	2602.54	22.41

BREAKFAST
Country Hash Browns and Egg Whites*, 1 serving
1 slice toasted multigrain bread
Light butter or 40% vegetable oil spread, 1 tablespoon
Grapefruit, ½

MORNING MINI-MEAL
Cottage cheese, low-fat with pineapple, ½ cup

LUNCH
Crabmeat Quesadillas*, 1 serving
Strawberries, fresh or frozen and thawed, 1 cup
Nonfat milk, 1 cup

AFTERNOON MINI-MEAL
Broccoli, raw, 1 cup of florets
Light mayonnaise, 1 tablespoon
Orange juice, 8 ounces

DINNER
Slim Sloppy Joes*, 1 serving
Tossed salad, 1½ cups
Salad dressing, diet French, 2 ounces
Frozen yogurt, low-fat, 1 cup
Brownie, Weight Watchers, 1

Substitute fresh fruit for dessert if desired. Add breast-feeding bonus foods (pages 60–62) as needed—see Chapter 4.

*See Chapter 9 for recipes.

Month 3: Thursday

CALORIES	PROTEIN (G)	CARBS (G)	FAT (G)	SAT. FAT (G)	CHOL. (MG)	SODIUM (MG)	FIBER (G)
1533.66	98.30	242.41	24.03	7.78	93.01	2015.80	18.54

BREAKFAST
French Toast*, 1 serving
Orange
Nonfat milk, 1 cup

MORNING MINI-MEAL
Cheddar cheese, low-fat, 1 ounce
Vegetable juice, V-8 low-salt, 1 cup

LUNCH
Beef barley soup, Progresso, 1 cup
Multigrain bread, 1 slice
Nonfat milk, 1 cup
Grapes, 10

AFTERNOON MINI-MEAL
Apple
Celery, 2 stalks
Light mayonnaise, 1 tablespoon

DINNER
No-Yolk Pasta with Tuna White Sauce*, 1 serving
Tossed salad, 1½ cups
Salad dressing, diet French, 2 ounces

Frozen yogurt, low-fat, 1 serving
Granola cookies, Health Valley, 3

Substitute fresh fruit for dessert if desired. Add breast-feeding bonus foods (pages 60–62) as needed—see Chapter 4.

*See Chapter 9 for recipes.

Month 3: Friday

DAILY TOTALS, ALL FOODS

CALORIES	PROTEIN (G)	CARBS (G)	FAT (G)	SAT. FAT (G)	CHOL. (MG)	SODIUM (MG)	FIBER (G)
1563.41	84.46	225.96	41.38	13.66	107.34	2268.62	17.29

BREAKFAST
Cheerios cereal, 1 cup
Banana, ½ medium
Nonfat milk, 1 cup

MORNING MINI-MEAL
Orange
Tortilla chips, Guiltless Gourmet, 1 ounce
Cheddar cheese, low-fat, 1 ounce

LUNCH
Minestrone soup, Healthy Choice, 1 cup
SnackWell's Classic Golden Crackers, reduced fat, 6
Nonfat milk, 1 cup

AFTERNOON MINI-MEAL
Plum

DINNER

Stir-fried Beef with Japanese Noodles*, 1 serving

Granola cookies, Healthy Valley, 3

Nonfat milk, 1 cup

Substitute fresh fruit for dessert if desired. Add breast-feeding bonus foods (pages 60–62) as needed—see Chapter 4.

*See Chapter 9 for recipes.

Month 3: Saturday

DAILY TOTALS, ALL FOODS

CALORIES	PROTEIN (G)	CARBS (G)	FAT (G)	SAT. FAT (G)	CHOL. (MG)	SODIUM (MG)	FIBER (G)
1534.95	84.85	215.08	29.49	6.33	101.87	2316.51	20.12

BREAKFAST

Blueberry Egg White Pancakes*, 1 serving

MORNING MINI-MEAL

Apple, cut into 8 slices

Peanut butter, chunky, 2 tablespoons, spread on apple

LUNCH

Tuna Salad Pita Sandwich*

Vegetable juice, V-8 low-salt, 8 ounces

AFTERNOON MINI-MEAL

Popcorn, Gourmet microwave light butter-flavored, 3 cups

DINNER

Garlic-Rosemary Chicken*, 1 serving

Asparagus spears, fresh or canned, ½ cup

Italian bread, 1-inch slice

Light butter or 40% oil vegetable spread, 1 tablespoon

Strawberries, fresh or frozen and thawed, ½ cup

Whipped cream, light, 1 tablespoon

Champagne—to celebrate getting your body back!

Add breast-feeding bonus foods (pages 60–62) as needed—see Chapter 4.

*See Chapter 9 for recipes.

WORKABLE WORKOUTS FOR MONTH 3

This month, extend your fitness walks to 45 minutes each session. If your baby gets impossibly fussy during a longer walk, break the walk up into two 20-minute sessions, or quit after 30 minutes. But aim for a vigorous 45-minute walk, since this duration will activate your cells to release fat and maximize cardiovascular benefits.

Increase intensity by walking faster, further, and up more hills than you did last month. During the peak of the walk, you should be in the top half of your target heart rate zone. The pace should feel "somewhat hard" to "very hard," but should never feel painful or make you breathless. Get out and walk at least four days a week, instead of three. You'll feel great and your baby will become a hardy little outdoors person.

FITNESS WALK REMINDERS

- Make sure baby is well buckled into his stroller.

- Dress yourself in suitably warm, flexible clothing. Dress your baby in comfortable layers and add a hat if it's even mildly cool—sweet little ears tend to get cold.

- Feed and diaper your baby beforehand, and bring extra liquid and snacks.

- Walk at a moderate pace for the first 5 to 10 minutes to warm up your muscles, then increase the pace. Slow it down for the last 5 minutes of the walk.

- Slow down or stop if you ever feel breathless or dizzy.

- Do the cool-down stretches on pages 118–20 after each fitness walk.

POWER UP YOUR STRENGTH TRAINING

At least twice a week, do the basic Supermom's Strength-Training Routine on pages 146–50 but increase the repetitions as described below. Use 5-pound weights and if these don't feel challenging, move up to 8-pound weights. The goal is to feel like you're working your muscles hard, but not have it feel painful.

SUPERMOM'S STRENGTH-TRAINING ROUTINE FOR MONTH 3

Strength-Training Warm-up
1 set

Squats
2 sets of 20 repetitions

Rows
Using hand-held weights (5–8 pounds), 2 sets of 20 repetitions

Push-ups
3 sets of 10 push-ups, bent-knee or traditional depending on your strength

Ab Crunches
2 sets of 20 repetitions (be careful not to strain your neck)

After Strength-Training Stretches
1 set

INDOOR EXERCISE ALTERNATIVES: FITNESS VIDEOTAPES

Even if you can't leave your baby to go to a class, you can sample a wide range of workouts right in your own living room, by using fitness videotapes. Experimenting with different routines will keep you from getting bored and stale, and also have an important training effect. You'll work different muscle groups and tone various areas of your body. You'll discover which forms of exercise you prefer and want to pursue. And you'll have something active to do with the baby on a rainy day. Do an exercise video once or twice each week.

If the little one is still fairly immobile, you can set him up in a carrier or bouncy chair to watch you work out. He'll be entertained by the music, by watching the people jump around on TV, and most of all by seeing you do strange and silly moves.

If your baby is starting to crawl, creep, or walk, it's not realistic to expect that he'll let you get through an hour-long videotape. If you have a baby-proofed room that is well equipped with toys, and a child who doesn't mind playing by himself, you might make it through a half hour. Then you can break for a bottle or whatever and come back for the second half later. Another approach is to select shorter videotapes that focus on either aerobics, muscle toning, or stretching, rather than the longer combination workouts. But if your baby is too active and demanding of your attention, you might have to wait for naptime so you can do the workout without constant interruption.

A variety of exercise tapes can be rented from a video store or borrowed from the library. It's always a good idea to try them out before buying, if possible. Once you're ready to buy, you can purchase videotapes at a store or order them from a catalogue or Web site. Some of my favorite choices are listed in the Resources section at the end of this book.

Many Web sites have search features that help you to find videotapes that suit your fitness goals and level. Most beginning and intermediate level tapes should be suitable, as long as you have no injuries or special conditions.

Let's look at the five major categories of exercise videotapes and their benefits.

POSTPARTUM EXERCISES

- Offer a gentle, safe pace if you haven't exercised for a while

- Target the areas of the body that have been most affected by pregnancy (such as abs)

- Some include your baby in the workout

AEROBICS

- Strengthen the heart and build cardiovascular endurance

- Provide maximum fat-burning potential

- Increase metabolism so calories are used more effectively throughout the day

- Decrease stress; can increase optimism and lift your mood

MUSCLE TONING/STRENGTH TRAINING

- Sculpt your body

- Target specific areas

- Increase lean muscles, resulting in better ability to burn calories

- Build strength and confidence

COMBINATION AEROBIC/TONING

- Build cardiovascular strength and stamina

- Burn fat

- Strengthen muscles

- Improve flexibility

- Elevate mood

STRENGTH, YOGA, AND RELAXATION

- Improve flexibility

- Relieve stress

- Reduce the potential for back pain and injury

Another benefit of learning yoga is that once you're familiar with the stretches and yoga poses, you can do them while playing with your baby on the floor. I spent many a happy hour stretching on the rug in the nursery as I watched Belinda learn to sit up, crawl, and stand. Of course once she was walking and talking, she'd always want me to "wake up" if I held a pose too long.

WORKABLE WORKOUT MONTH 3 ACTION STEPS

1. Increase the frequency, intensity, and duration of your fitness walks to four sessions of 45 minutes per week.

2. Do the Supermom's Basic Strength-Training Routine twice a week; gradually increase the repetitions.

3. Pick out a selection of fitness videotapes to expand your exercise repertoire, and do a routine once or twice a week.

MOMMY CARE

You've been eating for energy and exercising regularly for over two months now. But if your darling baby still wakes you up during the night to nurse, bottle-feed, or retrieve the precious teddy bear that has fallen out of the crib, you might still be exhausted. What can you do to finally feel rested?

TAKING A TWENTY-MINUTE RELAXATION NAP

Interestingly, sleep researchers have found that a nap of a mere 20 minutes actually rejuvenates more than a longer nap (although it's human nature to want to sleep longer). When you're at home, the obvious time to take a nap is when the baby is napping, assuming you're close enough to hear her cry or you have a reliable baby monitor.

If you're at work all day, it's trickier. One idea is to nap on the bus or train when you're commuting home, provided you have a seatmate to wake you at your stop. Another possibility, if you have a private office or lounge, is to keep an exercise mat at work, and sneak in a little nap during lunchtime. Don't scoff—John D. Rockefeller, the patriarch who made the family fortune, was reported to take five naps a day, and look how much he accomplished. Of course, he had a nanny or two to take care of the babies.

THE TWENTY-MINUTE RELAXATION NAP ROUTINE

Here's how to get the maximum value out of limited naptime.

Loosen your clothing and turn off the lights or pull down the shade. If you have no essential business calls expected, turn off the phone. If you're at home and the baby's sleeping, you might want to let nature take its course. Otherwise, set a timer or alarm clock for twenty minutes.

Lie down on your back, with just one flat pillow, so that your spine can lengthen and relax. Breathe slowly into your abdomen for a count of 6. Exhale slowly for a count of 6. Do this a few times. Let your feet relax and your heels sink into the bed. Relax your legs. Relax your hips. Breathe into your abdomen. Exhale and let your muscles go. Relax your waist. Breathe into your chest, feeling your shoulder blades open up wide, then relax. Relax the tops of your shoulders. Let your arms feel heavy and warm. Relax your neck. Completely let go and sink into the pillows.

At this point, you might drift off into a relaxing cycle of sleep. If you don't, concentrate on deep, rhythmic breathing and the warm, relaxed feeling of your body. You'll find that a total relaxation period can be just as rejuvenating as actual sleep.

FALLING BACK TO SLEEP IN THE MIDDLE OF THE NIGHT

You gratefully fall asleep the minute you hit the pillow at bedtime, but a few hours later, the baby jolts you awake with the familiar sound of crying. You get up, give him a breast or bottle, rock him a little, and he falls back to sleep easily. You place him back in the crib, marvel at his perfection, and head back to your own bed, eager for more rest. But now, with the edge of your fatigue dissipated by a few hours' sleep and the sleep cycle interrupted, you can't regain unconsciousness. You toss and turn, then feel exhausted the next day.

Falling asleep is rarely an issue for honestly exhausted new moms. But falling *back* to sleep can be. Here are a few suggestions on overcoming this problem:

- Keep the lights dim when you feed the baby in the middle of the night. Close your eyes and relax as you feed him, so you keep that half-asleep feeling.

- Since caffeine can stay in your system for up to 12 hours, avoid caffeinated beverages (including sodas) in the evening.

- Drinking alcohol can also interfere with your ability to fall back asleep. Avoid it if you tend to have trouble sleeping after drinking.

- Use the deep breathing and body relaxation sequence described with the 20-minute relaxation nap (page 176) to help yourself drift back to sleep in the middle of the night.

- Try not to allow yourself to think about problems, worries, and responsibilities when you're lying in your bed. If you find yourself drifting into anxiety-provoking thoughts, turn your mind to your baby's face, his soft cheek, his delicious smell.

- Don't succumb to the temptation to take your baby into your bed in the hope of a better night's sleep. Once you adopt this habit, it's hard to get baby accustomed to sleeping in his own crib or bed.

- If you're tossing and turning anyway, consider waking up your partner for lovemaking. It's an opportunity to fit sex into a busy schedule and a great way to get back to sleep.

FINDING TIME FOR LOVEMAKING

Since you're slimming and toning and bursting with vitality by this third month of the program, you'll probably have a rekindled interest in sex. But when will you ever have a private moment?

It's an amusing paradox that the very act that creates babies is then inhibited by their presence. Perhaps you preferred to make love in the morning, but that's out, since baby is awake before the birdies at dawn. Or you liked to make love before going to sleep, but now you're so tired it seems like a chore. It's not easy to be a new mommy *and* a lover. Still, love will find a way.

One summer evening I saw a couple who are close friends of ours driving home without their one-year-old. They stopped to say hello and said they had just dropped off the baby at her grandma's for the evening and were so excited because they were going to have a night alone. When I asked where they were going, the wife gave a big smile and said, "Home."

It's an excellent idea. If you can leave your baby at a relative's house for an evening of babysitting, you don't necessarily have to head to a crowded movie theater or restaurant. It might be more satisfying to go home and have a date in bed.

Another possibility is the afternoon delight. If it's a weekend or a day when you're both home from work, don't waste the baby's naptime doing the laundry. Invite your husband to take a nap with you and seduce him in the middle of the day. Take advantage of the years when your baby is still young enough to be safely ensconced in a crib. Soon she'll be free to toddle all over the house and it will be even harder to find privacy.

AFTER PROGRAM REWARDS

When you've reached the end of the three-month program, step back to review your progress. First, put on the exact same outfit you wore for your preprogram portrait. Look in the mirror and compare. You'll probably notice a gratifying difference.

If you want more affirmation, take your measurements and compare them with the Preprogram Record. Keep in mind, however, that you've gained muscle as you've lost fat, so the scale doesn't tell the whole story.

After-Program Record

Weight (upon waking)_____

Chest (across bust)_____

Waist_____

Hips (widest point)_____

Thighs (widest point)_____

Dress size_____

Pant size_____

Preprogram weight_____

Prepregnancy weight_____

Desired weight _____
(If different)

Treat yourself to a little shopping trip as a reward for finishing the program. Buy something that shows off your new figure. Indulge in a dress that's wilder than your usual style. Don't worry if you have nowhere to wear it; you can model it at home. Or perhaps you want to try a new swimsuit, one of those attractive two-pieces that you couldn't wear last summer. Or a pair of leather pants. Or a fantasy lingerie outfit. Whatever it is you secretly desire, buy it, flaunt it, and know you deserve it.

Of course, any new outfit is trivial compared to the real reward: how much better you look and feel. The pride you get from having your body back. Your increased confidence in your will and strength. The sense of power you feel from accomplishing your goals. The patience, energy, and sheer joy in life that you have to share with your baby.

CHAPTER 9

THE **HELP** SIMPLE AND SATISFYING RECIPES

The recipes are grouped into three categories: breakfast, lunch and mini-meals, dinner entrées, side dishes and dessert. Within these categories the recipes are listed alphabetically by title.

If the number of servings in the recipe is not appropriate for your circumstances, feel free to adjust it. For example, some lunches are for one person only, but if you have company you can double the ingredients. Most dinners are for four, which may be too much for your family size—although be forewarned that your husband will probably want two portions, unless he's also interested in slimming. Of course, you can always freeze leftovers.

Please be aware that the size of one serving is likely to be substantially smaller than what you're accustomed to eating. In some cases, it may be half the size of your usual portion. Sorry, but these smaller portions are a key to weight loss! If your spouse or other family members want larger portions, let them help themselves. But it is important that you measure out your portion and stay with the modest amount.

You will need a set of measuring cups, measuring spoons, and a food scale to measure ingredients and servings. A basic set of pots and pans including a nonstick pan, plus a toaster oven, microwave oven and blender will suffice. Lists of ingredients needed for each month of the program are found with the menu plans in Chapters 6 through 8.

BREAKFASTS

Apple-Cinnamon Grapefruit

1 large grapefruit
1 fluid ounce apple juice
⅛ teaspoon ground cinnamon

1. Cut the grapefruit in half and use a knife to loosen the segments. Spread the apple juice evenly on the grapefruit and sprinkle with cinnamon. Place on nonstick baking pan.

2. Broil for several minutes, until lightly browned.

SERVINGS: 2 (SERVING SIZE, ½ GRAPEFRUIT)   CALORIES/SERVING: 77.03

Blueberry Egg White Pancakes

4 egg whites or 8 ounces egg product (Egg beaters)
⅓ cup H-O whole grain instant oatmeal
2 tablespoons dried pancake mix
¼ cup low-fat buttermilk
2 tablespoons blueberry preserves
¼ cup fresh blueberries
Canola oil spray
Reduced calorie pancake syrup

1. Place the first five ingredients into a blender. Blend until smooth. Stir the blueberries into the batter.

2. Preheat a nonstick skillet over medium heat and spray with canola oil spray. Spoon the batter onto the skillet in the size desired and cook until the edges are dry. Turn and brown the other side. Add a drizzle of light pancake syrup.

SERVINGS: 2   CALORIES/SERVING: 326.27

Country Hash Browns and Egg Whites

Canola oil spray
Frozen hash brown potatoes, 1 patty
4 egg whites or 8 ounces liquid egg product (Egg Beaters)
1 dash salt
2 tablespoons chopped onion

1. Spray a small nonstick skillet with canola oil spray. Add 2 table-spoons of water and set heat to medium low. Add the potato patty and cook until patty is brown on both sides.

2. Remove the potatoes to a plate. Wipe skillet with paper towel and spray again. Add the egg whites, salt, and chopped onions. Stir until the eggs are firm.

SERVINGS: 1   CALORIES/SERVING: 140.54

French Toast

4 ounces egg product (Egg Beaters)
⅙ cup nonfat milk
½ teaspoon ground cinnamon
½ teaspoon vanilla extract
4 slices white bread
Canola oil spray
2 tablespoons reduced calorie pancake syrup

1. Mix the egg substitute, milk, cinnamon, and vanilla in a shallow pan or bowl. Dip the bread in the batter mix. Coat both sides.

2. Cook the French toast in a nonstick pan coated with canola oil spray over medium heat until lightly brown.

3. Turn and brown the other side. Serve with a tablespoon of pancake syrup for each serving.

SERVINGS: 2 (SERVING SIZE, 2 SLICES)   CALORIES/SERVING: 216.60

Salsa Breakfast Scramble

Canola oil spray
⅛ cup extra-lean ham lunch meat, diced
⅛ cup fresh button mushrooms, chopped
⅛ cup onions, chopped
4 ounces liquid egg product (Egg Beaters)
1 English muffin, split in half
2 tablespoons mild salsa

1. Spray a nonstick skillet with canola oil spray and sauté the ham, mushrooms, and onion. Mix in the egg substitute and scramble.

2. Toast the English muffin. Place half the scrambled mixture on top of each muffin half. Spoon salsa on top to taste.

SERVINGS: 2 (SERVING SIZE, ½ ENGLISH MUFFIN)   CALORIES/SERVING: 143.90

LUNCHES AND MINI-MEALS

Chicken Salad Pita Sandwich

1 10-ounce can chunk chicken breast, drained and flaked
½ teaspoon lemon-pepper seasoning
1 tablespoon chopped onion
½ cup chopped celery
½ tablespoon mustard

6 ounces light mayonnaise
2 small whole wheat pitas

1. Drain water from canned chunk chicken and place in a small bowl. Sprinkle the chicken with lemon-pepper seasoning. Chill in the refrigerator for 20 minutes if needed.

2. Combine the seasoned chicken with the onion, celery, mustard, and mayonnaise. Mix evenly.

3. Cut pitas in half and stuff the chicken mixture into each of the pitas. Then warm the pitas in the microwave or toaster oven.

SERVINGS: 4 (SERVING SIZE, ½ STUFFED PITA)   CALORIES/SERVING: 204.16

Crabmeat Quesadillas

2 6-ounce cans crabmeat, drained
Canola oil spray
4 low-fat burrito-sized tortillas
4 tablespoons mild fat-free salsa
1 cup shredded low-fat cheddar cheese
Salsa, mild, to taste

1. Preheat the oven to 350°. Place the crabmeat in a bowl and separate with a fork.

2. Spray an oven tray or baking sheet with canola oil spray and place 2 tortillas flat in the tray. Spread 2 tablespoons of salsa evenly on each tortilla. Add the crabmeat, smoothing out any clumps. Top evenly with shredded cheese. Place the remaining 2 tortillas on top of each quesadilla and gently press together.

3. Bake for 5 to 6 minutes. Remove from the oven and let cool 1 minute. Cut into slices like a pizza. Serve with extra salsa on the side.

SERVINGS: 4   CALORIES/SERVING: 287.44

Deviled Eggs

3 eggs
2 ounces liquid egg product (Eggbeaters)
⅛ teaspoon celery salt
1 tablespoon reduced fat mayonnaise
1 tablespoon mustard
1 tablespoon sweet pickle relish
⅛ teaspoon paprika (optional)

1. Hard-boil the eggs (about 20 minutes in boiling water). Peel them and slice lengthwise. Discard the yolks.

2. In a covered medium nonstick saucepan, cook the egg substitute over low heat for 10 minutes without stirring. Turn off the heat and let stand for 10 minutes, then remove the egg substitute from the saucepan and allow it to cool completely.

3. Chop the cooked egg substitute finely and put it in a medium bowl. Add the celery salt, mayonnaise, mustard, and pickle relish. Blend well. Use a small spoon to fill the egg white halves with this mixture. Sprinkle with the paprika and refrigerate until ready to serve.

SERVINGS: 6 (SERVING SIZE, 1 FILLED EGG HALF)   CALORIES/SERVING: 16.67

Fruit Smoothie

½ cup strawberries, hulled fresh or frozen and thawed
4 fluid ounces apple juice
½ banana
1 cup nonfat frozen peach yogurt (or fruit flavor of your choice)

1. Put all ingredients in a blender and blend until smooth.

2. If you want to extend the mixture, add ½ cup of crushed ice and blend again until smooth.

SERVINGS: 2   CALORIES/SERVING: 146.84

Italian Grilled Cheese and Tomato Sandwich

Canola oil spray
2 slices Italian bread
1.5 ounces cheddar cheese, sliced
2 slices tomato

1. Spray a nonstick skillet with canola oil spray. Put 1 slice of bread in the skillet. Place the cheese and tomato on the bread and cover with other slice of bread.

2. Cook over medium low heat until brown on one side. Flip onto the other side and cook until brown.

SERVINGS: 1   CALORIES/SERVING: 241

Tuna Salad Pita Sandwiches

1 stalk celery, chopped
3 ounces liquid egg product (Egg Beaters)

1 tablespoon chopped onion
1 tablespoon sweet pickle relish (optional)
⅙ cup reduced-fat mayonnaise
1 12-ounce can tuna in water, drained and flaked
2 small whole wheat pitas

1. Combine the first six ingredients.

2. Cut the pita bread into halves and warm in the microwave or toaster oven. Stuff the pita halves with the tuna mixture.

SERVINGS: 4 (SERVING SIZE, ½ PITA)   CALORIES/SERVING: 102.35

Turkey Sandwich

1 tablespoon reduced-fat mayonnaise
Dab of mustard (optional)
2 slices multigrain bread
1 ounce sliced lean turkey breast
1 ounce sliced nonfat ham lunch meat (optional), or add another ounce turkey
1 leaf lettuce
1 slice tomato

1. Spread the mayonnaise, and mustard if desired, on the bread.

2. Put the turkey, ham if desired, lettuce, and tomato on one slice of bread and top with the other slice.

SERVINGS: 1   CALORIES/SERVING: 217.68

DINNER ENTRÉES, SIDE DISHES, AND DESSERT

Baked Pears au Chocolate

2 fresh pears, or 4 canned pear halves
1 ounce orange liqueur (optional)
4 chocolate-covered mints
4 tablespoons light whipped topping
1 teaspoon sugar
4 seedless grapes, green or red, 1 whole grape per serving on top of
*   whipped topping*
1 cup water

1. If you are using fresh pears, peel, core, and halve the pears. Simmer the pears, covered, in water with a little sugar for 6 minutes or until soft to the touch, then drain well. Or, start with 4 canned pear halves, drained. Place the drained pear halves on an ovenproof plate.

2. Preheat the oven to 375°. Sprinkle the pear halves with the liqueur (optional). Put one chocolate-covered mint on top of each pear half. Bake the pears for 10 to 15 minutes, until the chocolate is melted.

3. Remove from the oven and garnish with whipped topping and grapes.

SERVINGS: 4 (SERVING SIZE, ½ PEAR)   CALORIES/SERVING: 147.83

Breaded Fish Fillets

1 egg white
½ teaspoon ground basil

¼ cup Italian bread crumbs
¼ cup cornmeal
1 teaspoon lemon zest, grated
¼ cup white wheat flour
⅛ teaspoon salt
¼ teaspoon lemon-pepper seasoning
4 4-ounce fillets (orange roughy, flounder, fillet of sole, or cod)
Canola oil spray

1. Preheat the oven to 450°. Beat the egg white until frothy in a medium bowl. Combine the basil, bread crumbs, cornmeal, and lemon peel in a shallow bowl. In another shallow dish, combine the flour, salt, and lemon-pepper seasoning.

2. Dip the fish fillets into the flour mixture and coat both sides. Dip the covered sides of the fillet into the egg white. Coat the covered sides of the fillet with the bread crumb mixture.

3. Spray a shallow baking pan with canola oil spray. Lay the prepared fillets side by side. Bake for 6 to 12 minutes, until the fish flakes easily with a fork.

SERVINGS: 4   CALORIES/SERVING: 168.81

Chinese Rice

Canola oil spray
½ cup finely chopped onion
16 ounces nonfat chicken broth
1 teaspoon light butter
¼ teaspoon hot pepper sauce
1 tablespoon low-sodium soy sauce or light teriyaki sauce
2 fluid ounces sherry

⅔ cup white rice
1 ounce pine nuts

1. Coat a medium saucepan with canola oil spray. Over medium
heat, sauté the onion. Add the broth, butter, hot pepper sauce, soy
sauce, and sherry and bring contents to a boil.

2. Stir the rice into broth mixture, and stir for 30 seconds to prevent sticking. Cover the pan, reduce the heat to low, and simmer
until the rice is tender and the liquid has been absorbed (about 25
minutes). Remove from heat.

3. Stir in the onions and pine nuts and serve.

SERVINGS: 4   CALORIES/SERVING: 78.63

Comforting Mashed Potatoes

2 pounds white Russett potatoes
1 tablespoon light butter
⅔ cup nonfat milk
1 teaspoon black pepper
1 teaspoon salt

1. Peel the potatoes while whole, then cut into quarters.

2. Bring a large saucepan of water to a boil. Boil the potatoes until
soft (about 20 minutes), then drain.

3. Combine the cooked potatoes, butter, milk, pepper, and salt in
a large bowl and mash thoroughly. Add a little water if needed to
create a creamy consistency.

SERVINGS: 4   CALORIES/SERVING: 213.41

Couscous-Stuffed Peppers

4 *medium green bell peppers*
2½ *cups nonfat chicken broth*
1¼ *cups couscous*
2 *tablespoons olive oil*
2 *tablespoons grated Parmesan cheese*
1 *medium tomato, chopped*
Canola oil spray
2 *tablespoons bread crumbs*
Salt
Black pepper

1. Preheat the oven to 350°. Bring a large saucepan of water to a rolling boil. Meanwhile, core and de-seed the peppers. Blanch the peppers in the boiling water for 2 minutes. Remove the peppers, drain, and set aside to cool.

2. Bring the chicken broth to low boil in a medium saucepan. Add a few drops of the olive oil to the broth. Gently stir the couscous into the boiling broth. Continue stirring to prevent clumping. Turn off the heat and cover. Let stand for 5 minutes. Uncover and stir with fork to fluff the couscous.

3. Place the couscous in a mixing bowl. Add the grated cheese, remaining olive oil, and chopped tomato. Stir and mix thoroughly.

4. Spray the peppers and a small baking pan with canola oil spray. Stuff the couscous mixture into the peppers and place in the baking pan. Sprinkle with bread crumbs and the remaining olive oil. Bake for 25 to 30 minutes. Sprinkle salt and pepper to taste.

SERVINGS: 4   CALORIES/SERVING: 386.80

Garlic-Rosemary Chicken

1 tablespoon canola oil
1 pound chicken breast, skinless and boneless, cut into 4 pieces
¾ teaspoon garlic powder
¾ teaspoon dried rosemary
⅓ cup water
10.5 ounces low-sodium chicken broth
1 cup instant brown rice, uncooked

1. Heat the oil in a large nonstick skillet on medium-high heat. Add the chicken and sprinkle with ¼ teaspoon of the garlic powder and ¼ teaspoon of the rosemary. Cover and cook 4 minutes on each side, or until cooked through. Remove the chicken from the skillet and set aside.

2. Add the water and broth to the skillet, stir, and bring to boil. Stir in the rice and remaining garlic powder and rosemary. Cover.

3. Cook on low heat 5 minutes. Remove from the heat and let stand 5 minutes before serving.

Serve chicken on a bed of rice.

SERVINGS: 4   CALORIES/SERVING: 300.49

Grilled Glazed Pork Chops

4 4-ounce center loin pork chops
½ teaspoon black pepper
4 cloves garlic, minced
⅔ cup orange marmalade
2 tablespoons fresh peppermint, chopped
¼ cup low-sodium soy sauce or light teriyaki sauce

1. Preheat your barbecue grill or broiler.

2. Place the chops between two sheets of waxed paper and flatten them slightly with a meat mallet. Sprinkle the chops with pepper.

3. Combine the garlic with the orange marmalade, peppermint, and soy sauce in a small saucepan. Brush part of this mixture over the pork chops.

4. Grill (or broil) the pork chops about 8 minutes per side. As you grill (or broil), baste frequently with the marmalade mixture.

5. Warm the remaining marmalade mixture over medium heat about 1 minute, and pour over the pork chops before serving.

SERVINGS: 4   CALORIES/SERVING: 304.11

Grilled Thai Ginger Tuna Steak

1½ pounds yellowfin tuna steaks, cut into 4 pieces
6 tablespoons low-sodium soy sauce or light teriyaki sauce
4 ounces white cooking wine
1 lime
3 tablespoons ground ginger
4 tablespoons garlic powder
1 teaspoon black pepper
Canola oil spray

1. Place tuna steaks on a large plate and coat with soy sauce, wine, and the juice of ½ of the lime.

2. Sprinkle garlic, ginger, and pepper over the steaks. Let marinate for 5–30 minutes.

3. Preheat the grill or broiler 5 minutes before cooking. Spray the tuna steaks and the grill or broiling pan with canola oil spray.

4. Cook 3 minutes on each side if grilling; cook 3–4 minutes per side if broiling. Remove when slightly crisp on top. If broiling fish pour the remaining marinade over the steaks in the broiling pan. If grilling you may baste the steaks with remaining marinade. Discard any leftover marinade. Garnish steaks with lime wedges cut from the remaining half lime.

SERVINGS: 4   CALORIES/SERVING: 333.78

Italian Grilled Tomatoes

2 whole large tomatoes
¼ teaspoon black pepper
1 teaspoon dill weed
½ ounce grated Parmesan cheese
½ ounce shredded mozzarella cheese
Canola oil spray

1. Preheat the broiler. Cut the tomatoes in half and place in a baking pan sprayed with canola oil. Sprinkle the tops of the tomatoes with pepper and dill weed and top with the cheeses.

2. Spray the tomatoes lightly with canola oil. Broil for 6 to 8 minutes.

SERVINGS: 4 (SERVING SIZE, ½ TOMATO)   CALORIES/SERVING: 35.08

Lamb Chops with Shallots and Red Wine

8 loin lamb chops, trimmed to ¼-inch fat
4 ounces red table wine

2 tablespoons vegetable oil
¼ cup chopped shallots
1 teaspoon dried rosemary
¼ teaspoon ground thyme
¼ teaspoon salt
¼ teaspoon black pepper

1. Nick the edges of the chops in several places to prevent curling. Place the chops in a baking dish.

2. In a small bowl whisk together all the other ingredients. Pour the mixture over the chops and cover. Marinate in the refrigerator at least 2 hours, turning once.

3. Remove the chops and discard the marinade. Let the lamb come to room temperature before grilling.

4. Preheat your grill or broiler. Cook 3 to 5 minutes per side, turning once.

SERVINGS: 4   CALORIES/SERVING: 277.14

Lean Turkey Burgers

½ cup chopped onion
½ cup chopped celery
3 cups water
1 pound extra-lean ground turkey
1 teaspoon horseradish
1 teaspoon low-sodium soy sauce or teriyaki sauce
¼ teaspoon salt
2 dashes black pepper
½ teaspoon garlic powder

½ teaspoon dried parsley
4 egg whites
Canola oil spray
4 whole wheat hamburger buns
4 lettuce leaves
4 tomato slices
Ketchup and mustard to taste

1. In a small saucepan, boil the onion and celery together in the water for 5 minutes. Drain and puree.

2. In a large bowl combine the puree with the turkey, horseradish, soy sauce, salt, pepper, garlic powder, parsley, and egg whites. Mix thoroughly and form into 4 patties.

3. Spray your grill or skillet lightly with canola oil spray. (Safety hint: Never leave sprays on or near the grill or stove.) Cook the burgers for 5 to 6 minutes on each side, or until well done. Turkey must be cooked thoroughly with no pink in the center of the burger.

4. Place each burger into a whole wheat bun. Top each with a lettuce leaf, a tomato slice, and ketchup and mustard to taste.

SERVINGS: 4   CALORIES/SERVING: 255.98

Low-fat Fettucine Alfredo

½ pound whole wheat fettucine pasta
¼ pound fresh button mushrooms
3 cloves garlic, minced, sliced
1 cup chopped onion
1 teaspoon Italian seasoning
½ teaspoon ground basil

⅛ *cup white wine*
½ *cup water*
1 *teaspoon onion powder*
⅛ *teaspoon black pepper*
3 *ounces evaporated milk*
1½ *cups small-curd low-fat cottage cheese*
1 *tablespoon whole wheat flour, presifted (or sift before use)*
½ *cup chopped fresh parsley*
½ *tablespoon garlic powder*
2 *dashes nutmeg*

1. Sauté the mushrooms, garlic, onion, Italian seasoning, basil, and white wine in a large frying pan until the liquid is absorbed. Set aside.

2. Cook and drain the fettucine.

3. In a medium nonstick saucepan, combine the water, onion powder, pepper, evaporated milk, and cottage cheese. Add the flour gradually, while stirring, and bring the mixture to a boil. Cook for 5 minutes, stirring frequently.

4. Toss the pasta, sauce, and sautéed mushroom mixture together and heat for 5 minutes. During the last 30 seconds, stir in the parsley, garlic powder, and nutmeg.

SERVINGS: 4   CALORIES/SERVING: 334.69

Marinated Flank Steak

1 *pound beef flank*
¼ *teaspoon garlic powder*
⅛ *teaspoon hot pepper sauce*

½ teaspoon onion powder
1 teaspoon ground thyme
4 ounces red wine vinegar
6 teaspoons Worcestershire sauce

1. Prepare the marinade by mixing all ingredients except the steak together. Put the marinade in a sealable freezer bag with the steak. Marinate in the refrigerator for 1 hour or more.

2. Remove the steak from the bag. Preheat your grill or broiler. Cook 3 to 4 minutes per side. (Flank steak becomes tough if cooked too long.) Slice across or against the grain to make it more tender.

SERVINGS: 4   CALORIES/SERVING: 188.64

Mom's Turkey Meatloaf

1 cup chopped onion
1 pound ground turkey
4 egg whites
½ teaspoon garlic powder
4 ounces multigrain oatmeal
2 dashes black pepper
8 ounces mild salsa
1 envelope Lipton Spring Vegetable soup mix
½ cup ketchup

1. Preheat the oven to 350°

2. Mix all the ingredients except the ketchup in a large bowl until well blended and form into loaf.

3. Spray a 9 × 5 baking pan with canola oil.

4. Place meatloaf in and gently press loaf to conform with pan.

5. Cover the top of the meatloaf with ketchup. Bake for 1½ hours.

SERVINGS: 6   CALORIES/SERVING: 164.84

No-Yolk Pasta with Tuna White Sauce

2 tablespoons light butter or 40% vegetable oil spread
12 ounces tuna canned in water, drained and flaked
1 large tomato, chopped
½ cup 2% fat milk
1 tablespoon ground basil
3 dashes salt
1 teaspoon black pepper
4 tablespoons grated Parmesan cheese
1 tablespoon garlic powder
8 ounces no-yolk egg noodles
4 quarts water

1. Melt the butter in a medium saucepan. Add the tuna and tomato. Sauté for 2 to 3 minutes.

2. Add all the remaining ingredients except the pasta. Cook and stir. Let simmer and stir about 2 minutes. Reduce the heat to low to keep warm.

3. Meanwhile, boil the water in a large pot. Cook the pasta 8 minutes. Drain the pasta, put into a serving dish, and spoon the sauce over the top.

SERVINGS 4   CALORIES/SERVING: 363.47

Savory Tarragon Chicken

1 *pound of boneless chicken breasts divided into 4 equal pieces, skin removed*
¼ *teaspoon mustard powder*
4 *tablespoons orange juice*
¼ *teaspoon parsley flakes*
¼ *teaspoon ground tarragon*

1. Place the chicken on a broiler pan. Combine the remaining ingredients in a bowl and mix well. Brush half the mixture over the chicken.

2. Broil for 6 minutes, or until lightly browned. Turn the chicken and brush the other side with the remaining herb mixture. Broil for 6 minutes more, or until the chicken is tender.

SERVINGS: 4   CALORIES/SERVING: 99.16

Seasoned Stuffed Potatoes

2 *large white Russet potatoes*
¼ *cup chopped onion*
4 *tablespoons water*
1 *egg white*
⅔ *cup low-fat buttermilk*
1 *teaspoon mustard*
¼ *teaspoon dill weed*
⅓ *teaspoon onion powder*
⅓ *teaspoon garlic powder*
⅙ *teaspoon horseradish*
1 *tablespoon grated Parmesan cheese*
1 *teaspoon dried parsley, ground*
⅓ *teaspoon paprika*

1. Preheat the over to 350°. Poke holes in the potatoes with a fork to release steam, then bake for 1 to 1½ hours or until tender. Leave oven on after removing potatoes.

2. Sauté the onion in a few tablespoons water. Beat the egg white until stiff.

3. Cut the baked potatoes in half lengthwise and scoop out the insides with a spoon. Save the skins intact for stuffing. In a large bowl whip the potatoes with the buttermilk, mustard, parsley, dill weed, onion powder, garlic powder, horseradish, grated cheese, and sautéed onions. Fold in the egg whites last. Stuff the potato skins with the mixture.

4. Place the stuffed potatoes in a nonstick baking pan, and sprinkle with paprika and parsley. Bake until hot and browned, about 15 minutes.

SERVINGS: 4 (SERVING SIZE, ½ POTATO)   **CALORIES/SERVING: 109.69**

Slim Sloppy Joes

1 pound ground turkey
6 teaspoons Butter Buds Sprinkles
¾ cup low-salt ketchup
½ cup diced celery
½ teaspoon mustard
¼ cup chopped onion
2 tablespoons brown sugar
3 tablespoons red wine vinegar
3 tablespoons Worcestershire sauce
2 English muffins, split

1. Mix together all the ingredients except the English muffins in a nonstick skillet. Simmer the mixture for about an hour.

2. Lightly toast the English muffins. Spoon the sloppy joe mixture over the muffin halves.

SERVINGS: 4   CALORIES/SERVING: 277.67

Spaghetti and Modern Meatballs

½ cup finely chopped or diced onion
½ cup finely chopped or diced celery
1 pound ground turkey
2 egg whites
4 slices whole wheat bread, broken into crumbs
½ teaspoon garlic powder
1 tablespoon dried parsley
½ teaspoon black pepper
Canola oil spray
1 pound spaghetti pasta
13 ounces chunky garden-style spaghetti sauce
4 quarts water

1. In a small saucepan, boil the onion and celery together in the water for 5 minutes. Drain with slotted spoon. Save water for pasta.

2. In a large mixing bowl, combine the ground turkey, egg whites, bread crumbs, onion, celery, and spices. Form into meatballs about 2 inches in diameter.

3. Spray a large skillet with the canola oil spray. Sauté the meatballs for 10 to 15 minutes over medium heat, turning occasionally, until completely browned. Drain on paper towels.

4. Clean the skillet and spray again lightly with canola oil. Combine the meatballs and sauce and simmer over low heat for 10 minutes.

5. Meanwhile, boil the water in a large pot, cook the pasta 8–10 minutes and drain. Place pasta in serving dish and spoon the meatballs and sauce over the drained pasta.

SERVINGS: 6 (SERVING SIZE, 1 CUP PASTA AND 4 MEATBALLS)

CALORIES/SERVING: 195.62

Steak and Vegetable Kabobs

6 ounces beef top sirloin, cubed
2 tablespoons diet Italian dressing
1 cup mushrooms
1 cup sliced onion
1 large green bell pepper, cut into 2-inch squares
4 skewers
1 cup medium-grain instant brown rice, cooked according to package directions
Canola oil spray (optional)

1. In a plastic zip-close bag or covered dish, marinate the sirloin in the light Italian dressing for 1 hour or longer in the refrigerator.

2. Preheat your grill. Alternate the mushrooms, onions, and pepper with the sirloin cubes on the skewers and grill for 6 minutes, turning frequently. Serve on the rice.

3. VARIATIONS: Add additional vegetables such as zucchini or yellow squash if you wish. Instead of grilling, you can sauté the meat and vegetables in olive oil until done.

SERVINGS: 4 (SERVING SIZE, 1 SKEWER)   CALORIES/SERVING: 376.38

Stir-fried Beef with Japanese Noodles

3 quarts water
2 tablespoons extra-virgin olive oil
6 ounces traditional Japanese udon noodles
1 pound beef round, trimmed to ¼-inch fat and cut into 3-inch strips
½ cup grated carrots
3 tablespoons light teriyaki sauce
1 tablespoon Worcestershire sauce
½ teaspoon garlic powder
½ teaspoon ground ginger
4 ounces fresh shiitake mushrooms, chopped

1. Heat the water in a large pot and add 1½ tablespoon of the oil.
Bring to a boil on medium heat. Add the noodles. When boiling,
cook for 3 to 4 minutes, then drain.

2. Place the remaining 1½ tablespoons oil in a large skillet or wok
and heat on medium heat for 1 minute. Add all the rest of the
ingredients except the noodles. Stir and brown evenly on medium
heat for 3 minutes.

3. Add the noodles to the meat mixture. Stir-fry 1 minute.

SERVINGS: 4   CALORIES/SERVING: 560.48

Stuffed Chicken Breasts

1 cup finely chopped fresh tomato
1 cup spinach, fresh or frozen and thawed, thoroughly drained (if
    using fresh, wash, drain, and dry spinach, chop thoroughly, and
    measure 1 cup packed slightly)
1 teaspoon grated lemon peel zest
2 teaspoons light butter

3 teaspoons dried parsley
4 4-ounce boneless and skinless chicken breasts
½ cup dried Italian bread crumbs
Canola oil spray

1. In a bowl combine the tomatoes and spinach with the lemon peel, butter, and parsley.

2. Preheat the oven to 350°. Place the chicken breasts between two sheets of waxed paper and flatten slightly by pounding lightly with a meat mallet. Spread an equal portion of the tomato-spinach mixture over each of the chicken breasts. Roll up the chicken breasts and fasten with wooden toothpicks.

3. Place the bread crumbs on a plate and roll each breast in them.

4. Put the breaded breasts in a shallow baking pan that has been sprayed with canola oil. Spray chicken rollups lightly on top and bake 35 to 40 minutes. Remove the toothpicks when done.

SERVINGS: 4   CALORIES/SERVING: 208.73

Sweet Potato Puffs

2 medium sweet potatoes
1 fluid ounce orange juice
¼ teaspoon ground ginger
⅛ teaspoon ground nutmeg
2 egg whites

1. Preheat the oven to 350°. Bring a large saucepan of water to a boil. Peel and quarter the sweet potatoes, and place immediately into the boiling water. Boil the potatoes until soft, then drain them.

2. Mash the potatoes in a large bowl. Add the orange juice, ginger, and nutmeg, and combine. Let cool. In a separate bowl, beat the egg whites until stiff peaks form and fold them into the sweet potato mixture.

3. Spoon the potatoes into a nonstick baking dish (balls should be about 2 inches in diameter and 2 inches apart) and bake for 30 minutes.

SERVINGS: 4   CALORIES/SERVING: 115.61

Tangy Baked Dover Sole

4 4-ounce sole fillets
½ teaspoon salt
½ teaspoon black pepper
¼ cup bottled lemon juice
¼ cup orange juice
1 teaspoon cornstarch dissolved in 2 tablespoons water
1 orange, cut into sections

1. Lay the fish flat in one layer in a large baking dish sprayed with canola oil. Season with salt and pepper. Pour the lemon and orange juices over the fish and cover. Marinate in the refrigerator for 1 hour.

2. Preheat the oven to 425°. Remove the fish from the refrigerator and cover the dish tightly with foil. Bake 8 to 10 minutes, or until the fish is opaque throughout. Transfer the fish to warmed individual serving plates and cover with foil, reserving the liquid.

3. Pour the reserved liquid into a small saucepan. Stir the dissolved cornstarch into the liquid and bring to a boil over medium-high heat, stirring until thickened (about 1 minute).

4. Spoon the sauce over the fish and garnish with orange sections.

SERVINGS: 4   CALORIES/SERVING: 114.74

Veal Scallopini with Lemon-Caper Sauce

1 pound veal leg, sliced scallopini style
6 tablespoons light teriyaki sauce
2½ ounces white cooking wine
6 tablespoons Italian bread crumbs
6 tablespoons extra-virgin olive oil
8 cloves garlic, chopped
12 small fresh button mushrooms, sliced
4 tablespoons drained capers
2 lemons

1. Place the veal between two sheets of waxed paper and tenderize slightly with a meat mallet. Put the veal in a baking dish to marinate. Add the teriyaki sauce and white wine. Turn the veal to coat evenly and set aside.

2. Put the bread crumbs on a plate. Coat each slice of veal on each side with bread crumbs, and put onto another plate. Reserve the marinade.

3. Place the olive oil in a large skillet and heat on medium heat. When hot, add the veal, garlic, and mushrooms. Sauté until golden brown, then turn the meat and lightly brown other side, cooking about 2 minutes per side.

4. Sprinkle the capers and the juice of 1 lemon on top of the meat mixture. Add the reserved marinade. Reduce the heat and cook

for 1 minute more. Serve veal with the sauce spooned over it and a
lemon wedge for garnish.

SERVINGS: 4   CALORIES/SERVING: 422.73

Veggie Chili

1 16-ounce package vegetarian (meatless) burger mix
1 onion, chopped
1 cup chopped green bell pepper
3 cloves garlic, chopped
½ cup carrot strips
16 ounces canned crushed tomatoes
16 ounces canned tomato sauce
16 ounces canned kidney beans
2 tablespoons chili powder
¾ teaspoon cumin seed
¼ teaspoon cayenne pepper.

1. Following the package directions, make and cook four vegetarian burgers.

2. Combine the rest of the ingredients in a large pot. Crumble the
burgers with your fingers and add to the chili sauce. Simmer for 30
minutes. Stir occasionally to keep from sticking to sides of pot.

SERVINGS: 4   CALORIES/SERVING: 360.18

CHAPTER 10

KEEP YOUR BODY BACK:

Achieving and Maintaining Your Goals

For three months you've worked hard to stick to the diet plan and exercise schedule. You've seen rewarding results. But alas, you can't just rest on your laurels. Unless you're one of the rare and envied species of women known as "naturally thin," you need a strategy to stay fit in the face of endless temptations.

MAINTENANCE EATING

PORTION CONTROL

The reality is that any food, even low-fat choices, can add extra weight if you eat too much of it on a regular basis. Very often, we choose foods intelligently, but undermine our efforts by eating too much of a good thing.

To avoid this pitfall, become adept at practicing portion control. Here are the basic portion sizes that will help you lose the last few pounds, or at least maintain and not gain.

FOOD	PORTION
Meat, Chicken, Fish, or Tofu	3–5 ounces (3 ounces is the same size as the palm of your hand, a playing card, or a credit card)
Pasta	½ cup–1 cup, cooked (1 cup is the same size as your fist or a tennis ball; you need only half that much as a side dish)
Starchy Vegetables	½ cup, cooked
Fruit Juice	6 ounces
Vegetables	1 cup raw; ½ cup cooked
Bread (that is not presliced)	1 slice the size of a CD jewel case
Fat (butter, oil, mayonnaise)	1 tablespoon (about the size of your thumb)
Cheese	1 ounce (a cube that measures 1 inch on each side)

These portion sizes are probably far less than you'd normally heap on your plate. Hopefully, the three months on the HELP for Moms plan have conditioned you to eating smaller portions. But it is always a struggle if you love to eat. It helps to drink a big glass of water before a meal. Put your food on a salad or lunch plate instead of a large dinner plate, so that the smaller portion doesn't look too measly. Eat slowly and chew thoroughly. And console yourself with the knowledge that with a smaller portion, at least you can finish before your baby interrupts the meal.

Keep in mind these sad but true facts about portions:

- A large "New York" bagel could be two or three "controlled" servings of bread

- A heaping bowl of cereal could be two to four servings

- A restaurant-size plate of pasta could be three to six servings!

MOTHER'S HELPER HINT: Keep ingredients for a fresh salad in your refrigerator at all times: lettuce, carrots, tomatoes, celery, raw cauliflower or broccoli, pre-washed lettuce and low-fat dressing. These are more expensive than heads of lettuce, but wonderfully convenient. Then, when you crave a heaping portion of *something*, have a big bowl of salad, with a light portion of nonfat dressing.

LOW-FAT EATING FOR LIFE

Since low-fat cooking is crucial for heart health as well as weight maintenance, there is a lot of information available on this topic. From down-home basics to low-fat versions of the diverse cooking cultures of the world, you can find a wealth of guides and recipes to suit your lifestyle and cooking expertise. There is also an abundance of material available on the Web.

Be aware that low fat does not mean no fat. Everyone can and should have a certain amount of dietary fat in their diet. And some forms of fat are certainly more harmful than others. Saturated fat from animal and dairy sources is a chief culprit when it comes to risk of cardiovascular disease and obesity. Trans fats or partially hydrogenated oils, which are found in many processed foods (especially baked goods) and fried fast foods, are also undesirable.

Essential fatty acids are generally considered "good" fats since they are utilized in many important body functions. They are found in egg yolks, cold-water ocean fish, nuts, soybeans, whole grains, canola oil, olive oil, and flaxseed oil. But when it comes to weight control, moderation is required whether or not a particular form of fat is "naughty or nice."

Here are some basic healthy, low-fat eating tips to keep in mind.

- Always keep two cartons of milk in your refrigerator: whole milk for your baby or toddler; skim milk or 1% milk for you. Don't make the mistake of drinking whole milk because you have it in the house to plump up the baby.

- Select low-fat or fat-free cheeses. Be wary of cheese; a little is a lot.

- Choose low-fat versions of condiments such as butter, mayonnaise, and salad dressings.

- Keep sorbet or frozen yogurt in your freezer for a dessert treat instead of ice cream.

- Try soy or low-fat turkey breakfast meats instead of the traditional bacon or sausage.

- Look for baked pretzels and chips as snack foods instead of lard-fried chips.

- Buy lots of fresh fruits to satisfy your sweet tooth.

- Purchase lots of fresh vegetables, plus a good supply of frozen or canned vegetables.

- Have fresh salad ingredients available for an attack of the "munchies."

- Avoid doughnuts and croissants; use minimal butter on other breads.

- Buy a spice rack and stock it with flavorful spices for seasoning.

- Use canola oil, safflower oil, and olive oil or oil sprays instead of butter or lard for cooking.

- Choose extra-lean cuts of meat and poultry.

- Pick tuna canned in water instead of oil.

BETTER FOR YOU, BETTER FOR EVERYONE

It's very hard to control your eating if you have cookies, cake, candy, ice cream, chips, etc., in your house, lying in wait for a weak moment. Why not make it a permanent habit to keep your house free of these supertempting but sabotaging foods?

Perhaps your rationale is that you're buying these products for other members of your family. Step back a minute and consider. Who is really benefiting from foods that have low (or no) nutritional value? High-fat and sugary foods do not benefit anyone. If they're not in the house, your partner will be trimmer, healthier, and less prone to heart disease. Your children won't develop a sugar or junk food addiction, and they are less likely to have weight problems.

Before you buy sweets and junk food, ask yourself these questions: Who is going to eat it? Who needs it? Does it improve anyone's health, strength, or mood? Why should we eat it instead of healthy food?

If you answer these questions honestly, you might find that you're buying cookies for your husband, but you end up eating 80 percent of the box yourself in two days. Or you're buying candy for your kids, but the sugar makes them wild and ruins their appetites. Unless there is a holiday, a party, or another special occasion, everyone will survive, and even thrive, without junk foods. You don't have to banish goodies from your world forever. But if you turn these foods into occasional indulgences instead of standard fare you'll enjoy them more.

You'll be doing your children a favor if they become accustomed to healthy snacking. Kids can happily grow up snacking on fresh fruit, dried fruit, nuts, raw vegetables, and cereals. Sure, they may rebel when they're older and use their allowance money to buy candy bars. But they still have a better chance of developing healthy adult eating habits than if they get hooked on sugar in childhood.

Food Substitutions (to keep in mind at the supermarket)

FOOD	SUBSTITUTION
1. Bacon	Low-fat Canadian bacon; soy or low-fat turkey breakfast treat
2. Beer	Light beer
3. Biscuits	Fat-free biscuit mixes
4. Bologna	Sliced turkey or chicken breast
5. Butter	Light butter; 40% vegetable oil spread

FOOD	SUBSTITUTION
6. Cheese	Part-skim ricotta, cottage cheese; fat-free cheeses
7. Chocolate candy	Buy only a small nugget, not a bar
8. Chocolate pudding	Fat-free pudding
9. Coconut oil	Canola, safflower, sunflower, corn, or olive oil
10. Coffee creamer	Low-fat milk
11. Cookies	Graham crackers, animal crackers
12. Crackers	Fat-free crackers and bread sticks
13. Cream cheese	Fat-free cream cheese
14. Cream sauces for pasta	Marinara sauces
15. Danish	Half a cinnamon-raisin bagel
16. Eggs	Egg whites (or use one yolk for every two eggs); liquid egg product
17. Eggnog	Vanilla low-fat soy beverage
18. Gravy	Low-fat gravy, Worcestershire sauce
19. Ham	Turkey ham; nonfat 40% ham/water lunch meat

FOOD	SUBSTITUTION
20. Hamburger	Ground chicken or turkey
21. Hot dogs	Turkey or soy dogs
22. Ice cream	Sorbet, ice milk, or low-fat frozen yogurt
23. Juice w/fructose	Pure juice, mixed half and half with seltzer
24. Lard	Vegetable oils
25. Mayonnaise	Fat-free or low-fat mayonnaise
26. Meats	Soy-based meat substitutes
27. Muffins	Fat-free mixes
28. Nuts and seeds	Popcorn, pretzels
29. Oil	Nonstick cooking spray, olive and canola oil
30. Potato or tortilla chips	Baked chips
31. Salad dressings	Nonfat salad dressings
32. Sausage	Low-fat turkey sausages
33. Soda	Seltzer with a splash of fruit juice
34. Sour cream	Low-fat plain yogurt
35. Spaghetti sauce	Prepared low-fat spaghetti sauces

FOOD	SUBSTITUTION
36. Whipped cream	Vanilla-flavored nonfat or low-fat yogurt
37. Whole milk	Nonfat or low-fat milk
38. Wine	White wine spritzer

EATING OUT

By no means do you have to stay home measuring portions and counting calories to stay trim. Go out and enjoy yourself whenever you have a chance. Just think of all those stick-thin socialite "ladies who lunch" and Hollywood starlets who are always out on the town. With a little restraint and thoughtfulness, you can eat in restaurants and still stay in control.

Start off by skipping the bread. Without thinking, you can consume a whole dinner's worth of calories in bread and butter before the entrée arrives. If your dining companions don't want the bread, ask the waiter not to bring it. If they do, sip a white wine spritzer instead of attacking the bread basket.

Skip the appetizers. This will reduce the dollar cost of the meal as well as the caloric price. If you want two courses, have a salad.

Select dishes that are steamed, broiled, baked, roasted, poached, lightly sautéed, or stir-fried. Avoid dishes that are fried, creamy, or smothered in melted cheese.

Have cappuccino or an Irish coffee for dessert. Or share one dessert between two people.

Bring your baby. This will guarantee that you don't eat too much, unless she sleeps through the entire meal.

EATING OUT WITH YOUR BABY

When we started bringing Belinda to restaurants, we found that if we ordered appetizers, the statute of limitations on her sitting quietly ran out by the time the main course arrived. So we developed a strategy that allows for a peaceful meal:

- Pick a restaurant that prepares the food quickly—Chinese and Italian restaurants often do.

- Select a restaurant where people go to eat a satisfying meal, not to fall in love or celebrate a major milestone.

- Peruse the menu quickly and be ready to order your entrées when the waiter comes for your drink order.

- Skip the appetizers, and also the dessert—unless your baby is old enough to eat ice cream.

- Don't worry about the baby's eating a square meal at the restaurant. If she's content with a bottle, pacifier, or toy, or nibbling on a piece of bread, enjoy the peace. You can feed her more when you get home.

- Ask for the check as you're finishing your meal.

Leisurely dining with a baby or a toddler is an oxymoron. But if you use this strategic plan, you can make it out the door with everyone still cooing about how cute your baby is, instead of clucking with disapproval.

WORKING MOTHERS' LUNCHES

If you work outside the home, your most tempting meal might be lunch. It's practically the only chance you get to sit down for a meal without the baby interrupting. It's a welcome break from your hectic day and a chance to relieve stress. But you don't want it to be the meal that undermines your efforts to stay fit and trim.

Here are some tips for a lean but satisfying working lunch:

- Have a turkey sandwich instead of pastrami or ham.

- Order a grilled chicken breast sandwich instead of fried chicken.

- Use mustard, lettuce, pickles, and tomatoes to dress up your burger or sandwich instead of mayonnaise and cheese.

- Have a baked potato topped with a small amount of grated cheese, butter, or cottage cheese for a comfort meal.

- When you're at the salad bar, heap your plate with spinach, raw vegetables, and different types of lettuce. Go easy on the cheese, bacon bits, nuts, and seeds. Choose nonfat or low-fat dressing.

- Have a small cup of nonfat or low-fat frozen yogurt or a fruit cup for dessert.

- Be aware that even fat-free muffins can be huge and they are full of calories.

- Avoid a fast-food meal at any costs. They average 1200 calories and are not worth it!

AVOID THE TODDLER TEMPTATION TRAP

In the spirit of the shocking "tell-all" memoirs that have rocked the literary world, I offer up my own confession:

I have wolfed down macaroni and cheese shaped like "Blues Clues" characters.

I have polished off microwavable mini-meals of ravioli and beefaroni.

I have eaten leftover pudding cups brought by a devoted grandma to fatten up Belinda.

Once a baby is off the breast or bottle and on to solid food, a whole new world of temptation emerges. Unless you are blessed with the rare young child who finishes everything on her plate, you'll be facing a constant parade of leftovers. You will pack snacks in baggies for outings, only to be tempted to dip into them along the way. Well-meaning friends and relatives will give your darling child cookies, candies, cake, etc. During play dates you'll be confronted with bowls full of potato chips, tortilla chips, M&Ms. At luncheonettes, your child will lose interest in her grilled cheese sandwich and fries, leaving you with a dilemna—eat it or waste it.

Many mothers wouldn't dream of touching their children's leftovers or sharing their snacks. But there are also those of us who find ourselves consuming an unknown quantity of kiddie calories. It may be from frustration, if your child is a fussy eater. It may be boredom or sheer proximity. It may seem easier than fixing yourself something else to eat.

If you find yourself bedeviled by toddler temptations, take precautions. When you go on walks, let your child hold the snack and bring a water bottle for yourself. If you're tempted to munch on her snack, drink some water. When you embark on longer outings, bring fruit cut into small pieces instead of a bag of chips.

If you're on a play date, carry a bottle of water to sip. Bring a magazine to glance at if you think you'll have time on your hands. Have some popcorn, fruit, or crudité as a snack.

When you take your kids out for ice cream, order a small low-fat cup for yourself instead of "sharing" the premium brand. If you eat lunch out, order yourself a salad instead of consuming your kids' leftover hotdogs and chicken nuggets. Consider sharing a slice of pizza with a small child who doesn't eat a lot, instead of having your own slice *and* her leftovers.

Most importantly, establish a routine at home. If kids don't finish what's on their plate, you have two choices: save it or toss it. As soon as it's clear you can't coerce them to eat any more, store it in the fridge. If it's not worth saving, dump it in the garbage or give it to the dog. It will not save money if you eat it. It will not help underprivileged people who don't have enough food. And it certainly won't make your children grow bigger and stronger if *you* eat it!

GOOD FOR YOU, GOOD FOR THEM: SNACKS YOU SHOULD SHARE WITH YOUR KIDS

- Animal crackers, graham crackers, ginger snaps

- Peas in the pod (fun for children to open)

- Raw veggies, cut into fun shapes

- Pretzels

- Cheerios

- Tangerines and clementines

- Cored, pitted fresh fruits: apples, peaches, plums, pears, bananas

MAINTENANCE EXERCISE

WORK OUT WITH YOUR KIDS

When you're spending time with your children, be active as much as you can. It will lift your mood and reduce stress, plus provide an outlet for their boundless youthful energy.

OUTDOOR PHYSICAL ACTIVITIES

- Play tag, play ball, chase each other

- Garden or do yard work

- Go for short walks

- Stretch in the sun together; make it into a "Simon Says" game

- Keep moving when you're watching young children play together: pace, stretch, twist, jog in place

INDOOR ACTION

- Play "ballerina" by putting on dance clothes and dancing around to classical music

- Turn on your favorite rock music and dance

- Stretch and do yoga poses while playing on the floor

- Chase each other around the house

- Do strength-training exercises while watching the kids play.

CHILDREN'S EXERCISE VIDEOTAPES. Children's tapes are not as strenuous as grown-up fitness videos, but doing them with your child will get you moving. On a day when it's too cold or rainy for the playground, it's a great way to burn energy and have fun together. See the Resource Section for a selection of good videos for toddlers and older preschoolers.

ADJUSTING YOUR EXERCISE ROUTINE

Once your child is a toddler or preschooler, the golden age of fitness walks with the stroller will come to a close. Depending on his temperament, your child may or may not be willing to stay in the stroller long enough for you to gain any aerobic benefits. He may want to get up and walk, push the stroller, and career all over, so that walking becomes a game and no longer a workout. This is when you need to become more assertive about finding baby-sitting coverage so you can maintain your fitness gains.

The good news is that many health clubs, dance salons, and Ys have baby-sitting services available once your child is over the age of six months to one year. Baby-sitting is often provided for a nominal fee to encourage moms to participate. This offers a great opportunity for you to broaden your exercise horizons.

There's only one answer to the question of what the best form of exercise is. It's the one that you enjoy enough to keep doing. This is much more important than whether the workout burns 6 calories a minute or 16. Fun and pleasure are a huge incentive when it comes to exercise. The people who stay with it are the ones who find what they love to do.

You can choose from a wide scope of classes at health clubs, gyms, dance and martial arts schools, and Ys. Some current favorites:

- Aerobics: hip-hop, Latin, African, funk, step

- Kick-boxing, karate, kung fu

- Spinning

- Muscle toning, body sculpting, weight training

- Social dance: Latin, ballroom, country western

- Yoga, tai chi, Pilates

- Belly dancing, hula dancing, ballet dancing

Many people prefer to combine exercise with a chance to be outside in the fresh air. Outdoor exercise is free, it's invigorating, and it's often the best choice for life-long fitness. Walking, running, hiking, and biking are favorites. Swimming (outdoor or indoor) is both meditative and aerobic. Racquet sports, golf, and skiing are social and stimulating. As they said in the sixties: Follow your bliss.

FITNESS AND OLDER MOMS

Nature can play a funny trick on you if you have your baby later in life. The baby weight gain can meld seamlessly into weight gain from aging. You spend the first year or two thinking that it was childbirth that put on the pounds and thickened your waist. Then, as time marches on and so many other moms regain their figures, you realize that your lack of progress may be a sign of peri-menopause, not motherhood.

Researchers have found that virtually the only way to counter-act the weight gain and loss of muscle associated with aging is to combine increased exercise with careful diet. I wish I could offer an easier solution. But the reality is that if you have your babies in your late thirties or forties, you may have to work harder to get and keep your body back.

Here are some guidelines:

- Eat lightly at night

- Measure your fat intake and keep it under 25 percent of total calories

- Do aerobic exercise five times a week (or more) for 45 minutes per session

- Perform muscle-building/strength-training exercises a few times a week

WHEN YOU WANT TO LOSE MORE

What should you do if you're not satisfied with the results from your three months on The Get Your Body Back Program?

First, be sure that your goals are humane and realistic. Don't torture yourself by setting impossible standards. If you decide that you won't be satisfied unless you're a size 4, and you're not genetically inclined to be thin, you're setting yourself up for a lifetime of yo-yo dieting and self-recrimination.

How thin is thin enough? The answer is subjective and has many variables. That's why this book doesn't include the Metropolitan Life Table of Healthy Weights or other height/weight tables. These tables are ultimately meaningless. There are so many considerations when determining "ideal" weight: frame size and body type, muscle versus fat ratio, age, culture, even occupation.

Only you can decide what weight and level of toning are right for you. If you're in a design or fashion job or you're a performer, you may be pressured to be thinner than a "normal" person. If you love to wear skintight jeans and pencil skirts, you have different criteria than someone who's happy in loose flowing dresses. If you're athletic, you may weigh more because of muscle. If you're curvy and voluptuous, you'll look your best at a different size than someone with a boyish shape. Outside of being unhealthily obese, your ideal weight depends on your personal comfort level and predilections.

Honor your body and respect reality. Be kind to yourself by setting reasonable goals. Ask yourself these questions: What weight and dress size are you now? What would you like to be in an ideal world? What weight and size could you happily accept, even if they're not perfect? Who will care if you're the "acceptable" size instead of ideal? Will it affect your ability to be a good mother? A loving wife? Successful in your career? Comfortable with yourself?

Once you've answered these questions, write down:

My current weight and dress size:_____

My acceptable weight and dress size:_____

Now consider the difference between these two figures. If it is more than 5 pounds, you might want to continue the program for a month or two, with one difference: *Increase the intensity, duration, and frequency of your aerobic and strength-training exercise as much as you can.* Extra exercise is crucial. In addition to the calories used up by the exercise itself, the process of turning muscle into fat will raise your metabolic rate, enabling you to burn more calories throughout the day.

It is *not* recommended that you go below the basic 1500 to 1600 calories per day (plus up to 500 additional calories if you're breast-feeding full-time) in an effort to lose more pounds quickly. Research has determined that the faster weight comes off, the faster it is regained. And when you're a busy mom you can't afford to let your health or mood be compromised by a crash diet. Stay with a moderate eating program and increase your exercise to achieve your goals.

STAYING ON TRACK

If you face time constraints, temptations, and other obstacles, remember that *something* is always better than nothing when it comes to exercise and diet. Do as much as you can, but don't beat yourself up if you're not in perfect shape. With good grooming, flattering clothes, and a pleasant personality, you'll always be an attractive woman. Don't waste your life worrying about your weight.

Eat well so you have the fuel for your busy day. Exercise for the energy and the sheer pleasure of it. Take pride in your body and your accomplishments. Delight in being a healthy, joyful mommy—the most important person in the world to your family.

SELECTED RESOURCES

BOOKS

The choice of books on diet, nutrition, exercise, and advice for new mothers is so vast that you could spend the rest of your life reading about these topics. I often get lost at a mega-bookstore, browsing through the enticing titles in these areas.

Another great way to find books is to visit the Web sites of the major bookstores. You can browse on these sites while your baby is playing or resting, a nice way to expand your horizons while staying at home. These Web sites also offer a wide selection of exercise videotapes to suit every fitness level.

Here is a *very* selective list of books that are recommended if you want more information on some of the topics covered in this book:

American Heart Association. *The American Heart Association Cookbook*. Ballantine Books, New York, 1991. Over 500 low-fat recipes, most of which are low-calorie and easy to prepare.

Austin, Denise. *Lose Those Last Ten Pounds*. Broadway Books, New York, 2001. The peppy fitness queen offers an appealing 28-day program to burn off the last 10 pounds. A good choice if you want to reduce below your prepregnancy weight.

Behan, Eileen. *Eat Well, Lose Weight While Breastfeeding*. Villard

Books, New York, 1992. Although I'm not sure this book actually promotes weight loss, it does provide excellent advice on nutrition for women who are breast-feeding.

Eisenberg, Arlene, Heidi Murkoff, and Sandee Hathaway. *What to Expect the First Year*. Workman Publishing, New York, 1996. The authors of the classic *What to Expect When You're Expecting* deliver an immensely helpful book on not only caring for your baby, but caring for yourself during the first year.

Fischer, Lynn. *Lowfat Cooking for Dummies*. IDG Books Worldwide, Foster City, CA., 1997. Everything you need to know about low-fat cooking techniques, and lots of basic recipes.

Ridha, Arem, M.D. *The Thyroid Solution*. Random House, New York, 1999. Excellent advice on recognizing and treating thyroid disease, with an emphasis on the emotional symptoms of thyroid imbalance.

Ulene, Art, M.D. *The Nutribase Complete Book of Food Counts*. Avery Publishing Group, Garden City, NY, 1996. Calorie counts, plus protein, carbohydrate, sodium, fiber, fat, and cholesterol values for over 30,000 food items.

Waterhouse, Debra. *Outsmarting the Female Fat Cell*. Warner Books, New York, 1993. A very sensible, usable, and wise guide to losing fat and maintaining a life-long healthy weight.

Weight Watchers. *Simply Light Cooking*. New American Library, New York, 1991. Quick, easy, low-fat, and nutritious recipes.

EXERCISE VIDEOTAPES FOR MOMS

Denise Austin's Blast Off 10 Lbs. (Artisan), Aerobics/Toning, Intermediate Level. This videotape requires 2 to 5 pound dumbbells and 44 minutes of concentrated time, but pays off with a terrific workout. It starts off with cardio kickboxing (a good stress-reliever) and moves on to aerobics and toning.

Denise Austin's Bounce Back After Baby (Artisan), Postpartum, Beginning/Intermediate Level. This comprehensive workout includes 20 minutes of fat-burning aerobics, 15 minutes of toning/strengthening, and 10 minutes of relaxation exercise. Denise especially addresses the need to strengthen abdominal muscles if you've had a cesarean section.

Kathy Smith's Peak Fat-Burning (Sony), Aerobics, Intermediate Level. When you want to get serious about fitness, this 40-minute routine uses cardio interval training, which means intense 2-minute energy bursts followed by slower 2-minute movements.

Kathy Smith's Pilates for Abs (Sony), Pilates/Toning, Beginner/Intermediate Level. This videotape combines mat exercise inspired by J.H. Pilates with yoga moves in two 20-minute workouts. The exercises strengthen, lengthen, tone and stretch your muscles, leaving you relaxed and limber. Each workout is short enough to perform with your baby on the floor alongside you or watching from a comfy seat.

Leslie Sansone's Two Mile Walk (Parade Video), Aerobics, Beginner/Intermediate Level. This half-hour workout can replace your fitness walk on rainy days. Cheery Leslie Sansone keeps you going and the moves are simple enough to follow while cooing to your baby.

Richard Simmons Sweatin' to the Oldies Series (Warner Home Video), Aerobics, Beginner/Intermediate Level. Silly but fun, this series features aerobic workouts of about a half-hour duration with music that makes you want to move. The songs will get your baby dancing before she's walking.

Yoga Zone's Short Workout Series (Koch), Beginner, Yoga. There are two titles in this series: "Yoga Basics for Beginners" and "Power Yoga for Beginners." The Basics tape teaches you the proper form of classic poses, while the power yoga is faster and focuses on muscle toning. Each tape has two workouts of 18 minutes each, a feasible length when you have limited time.

EXERCISE VIDEOTAPES FOR YOUNG CHILDREN (AND THEIR MOMS)

A Fantasy Garden Ballet Class (Kultur): If you have a little girl who is over three and already taking dance classes, she'll adore this routine for pre-schoolers. The 40-minute class creatively uses flower and animal imagery to teach ballet steps. Mommy can get a mild workout and relive her childhood fantasies of being a ballerina if she dances along.

Elmocize (Sony): This half-hour show takes you to Elmo's Exercise Camp to bend, stretch, twist, and hop with the Muppets. There are lots of catchy tunes, such as "Workout in a Chair," and a guest appearance by pop star Cyndi Lauper, now a rockin' mama herself.

Sesame Street Get Up and Dance (Sony): Belinda calls this one "Dance with the Pretty Mommy" because it features a lovely dance instructor. The half-hour program is entertaining for both little kids and their parents. If you throw yourself into doing "the Airplane," "the Dog," and "the Jelly," you'll get a mild aerobic workout.

YogaKids (Living Arts): This lovely half-hour video includes twenty simple yoga poses, interspersed with songs, and nature clips. It requires more concentration than most toddlers can handle, but is provides a good stretching session for pre-schoolers and mommies.

DIET/FITNESS SOFTWARE

If you want to take the mystery out of dieting and find out the caloric and fat content of what you're eating each day, I recommend *Nutribase Nutrition and Fitness Software*. This excellent resource (which provided the basis for some of the recipes and meal plans in this book) essentially allows you to become your own expert nutritionist. You can access all the nutritional values of your daily intake, find ready-to-use low-fat meal plans and recipes, and create your own recipes. You can also track the caloric expenditure of your workouts and come up with a personalized fitness plan. Visit the Web site at nutribase.com or call 1-877-945-0315.

WEB SITES

If you type in key words such as "diet," "nutrition," "fitness," or "exercise," an Internet search will yield a bumper crop of Web sites on every imaginable topic. A few of my favorites:

- *ivillage.com*: The health link offers articles on nutrition, dieting, exercise, and stress reduction, many of them by top experts.

- *oxygen.com*: The thriveonline section of this Web site for women has helpful articles and features on fitness, nutrition, sexuality, and serenity.

- *weightwatchers.com*: Articles and low-fat recipes, also information on local Weight Watchers programs.

- *webmd.com*: Solid information on emotional and physical health issues.